# NURSING BEFORE NIGHTINGALE, 1815–1899

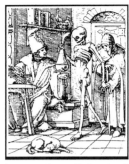

The History of Medicine in Context

Series Editors: Andrew Cunningham and Ole Peter Grell

Department of History and Philosophy of Science
University of Cambridge

Department of History
Open University

Titles in this series include

*Henri de Rothschild, 1872–1947*
*Medicine and Theater*
Harry W. Paul

*The Anatomist Anatomis'd*
*An Experimental Discipline in Enlightenment Europe*
Andrew Cunningham

*Centres of Medical Excellence?*
*Medical Travel and Education in Europe, 1500–1789*
Edited by Ole Peter Grell, Andrew Cunningham and Jon Arrizabalaga

*Ireland and Medicine in the Seventeenth and Eighteenth Centuries*
Edited by James Kelly and Fiona Clark

*Negotiating the French Pox in Early Modern Germany*
Claudia Stein

*Before My Helpless Sight*
*Suffering, Dying and Military Medicine on the Western Front, 1914–1918*
Leo van Bergen

# Nursing before Nightingale, 1815–1899

CAROL HELMSTADTER

JUDITH GODDEN

## ASHGATE

Published by
Ashgate Publishing Limited
Wey Court East
Union Road
Farnham
Surrey, GU9 7PT
England

Ashgate Publishing Company
Suite 420
101 Cherry Street
Burlington
VT 05401-4405
USA

www.ashgate.com

**British Library Cataloguing in Publication Data**
Helmstadter, Carol.
  Nursing before Nightingale, 1815-1899. -- (The history of
  medicine in context)
  1. Nursing--Great Britain--History--19th century.
  I. Title II. Series III. Godden, Judith.
  610.7'3'0941'09034-dc22

  ISBN-13: 9781409423133


**Library of Congress Cataloging-in-Publication Data**
Helmstadter, Carol.
  Nursing before Nightingale, 1815-1899 / Carol Helmstadter and Judith Godden.
     p. cm.
  Includes bibliographical references and index.
  ISBN 978-1-4094-2313-3 (hardcover) -- ISBN 978-1-4094-2314-0 (ebook)  1. Nursing-
-Great Britain--History--19th century.  I. Godden, Judith. II. Title.
  RT11.H45 2011
  610.73--dc23

                                                                        2011015342

ISBN 9781409423133 (hbk)
ISBN 9781409423140 (ebk)

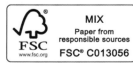

Printed and bound in Great Britain by
TJ International Ltd, Padstow, Cornwall.

# Contents

# List of Figures

# Note on Authors and Contributor

**Carol Helmstadter** is a retired neurosurgical nurse. She holds degrees in both history and nursing, and is also skilled in labour relations, having worked seven years as Government Relations Officer for Ontario Nurses Association. She is a past President of the Canadian Association for the History of Nursing, and has published widely on both clinical nursing and the history of nursing in nineteenth-century England. In 2008 the Canadian Nurses Association named her a Centennial Nurse for her contributions to nursing history.

**Judith Godden** is a professional historian and Honorary Associate at the Department of History, University of Sydney. She completed the early stages of this work as Senior Lecturer at the School of Public Health, University of Sydney. Judith is a past President of the Australian and New Zealand Society for the History of Medicine. She was awarded a C.H. Currey Memorial Fellowship from the State Library of New South Wales to write *Lucy Osburn, a Lady Displaced: Florence Nightingale's Envoy to Australia* (Sydney University Press, 2006), which was short-listed for Australia's 2008 National Biography Award. Her latest book is *Australia's Controversial Matron: Gwen Burbidge and Nursing Reform*, published by The College of Nursing, Sydney.

**Joyce Schroeder MacQueen** is a retired Associate Professor of Nursing at Laurentian University, Canada. She holds a degree in history as well, and has just completed a major oral history project on public health nursing in a Northern Canadian mining town. She has worked extensively on the Nightingale papers, in particular those dealing with her religious views.

# Preface

Investigations into the origins of modern nursing have been dominated by nursing politics and, more recently, a concern to correct past excesses. Initially, one narrative held sway: that nurses were callous, dirty and immoral until the second half of the nineteenth century, when they were replaced by younger, idealistic professional nurses. The prime reason given for the change was one woman: Florence Nightingale. She established, so the narrative went, the Nightingale system of training characterized by strict discipline under the ultimate control of a matron, a belief that nursing was first and foremost a vocation for women to care unselfishly for the sick, and that nurses should be unquestionably obedient to more senior colleagues and doctors. The older untrained nurses were branded 'Sarah Gamps' after the caricature of the callous domiciliary nurse created by the novelist Charles Dickens.[1] The fact that this historical interpretation reinforced the drive – almost monomania – of early twentieth-century nurses to be acknowledged as professionals with a similar status to that of doctors meant that this version of the great change in nursing was taught as the dominant narrative to generations of nurses. Admiring biographies of Nightingale reinforced the narrative.[2]

There had to be a reaction. It came in the 1980s, that 'astonishing decade of revision and critique of the traditional nursing narrative'.[3] In numerous works, Monica Baly deftly skewered the myth of the ultra-successful Nightingale School of Nursing at St Thomas' Hospital, the school portrayed as embodying Nightingale's ideals and credited with the worldwide spread of the new nurses.[4] New works questioned virtually every aspect of the old narrative, which Celia Davies condemned as 'largely congratulatory' and as selectively using evidence

---

[1]  Charles Dickens, *Martin Chuzzlewit*, first published in 1843–44. Gamp was almost immediately identified with hospital nurses.

[2]  Two foundational books for this dominant school of nursing history were Sarah Tooley, *The History of Nursing in the British Empire* (London, 1906), and M.A. Nutting and L.L. Dock, *A History of Nursing* (4 vols, New York, 1907–12). The most popular of the older Nightingale biographies was C. Woodham-Smith, *Florence Nightingale 1820—1910* (London, 1950).

[3]  S. Nelson, 'The Fork in the Road: Nursing History Versus the History of Nursing?', *Nursing History Review*, 10 (2002): pp. 175–88.

[4]  See, for example, M.E. Baly, *Florence Nightingale and the Nursing Legacy* (2nd edn, London, 1997).

to document recent nursing history solely 'as progress out of the dark ages to the present'.[5]

Crucially for the argument of this book, Anne Marie Rafferty and others pointed out that the change from the old to the new nurse was much more prolonged than previously thought, and that the bulk of the new nurses had much in common with the old nurses.[6] This challenge to the concept of a sharp break between the old and new nurses is still being taken up by nursing historians. Sue Hawkins is among the latest to reveal that the 'new' nurses were from a range of backgrounds and had similar concerns both to previous nurses and the rest of the workforce.[7] Our research offers further evidence that change in nursing did not represent a sharp break, but was a prolonged and difficult process.

The new nursing history from the 1980s was a child of its times; nurses saw parallels in new feminist interpretations of history, particularly that of midwifery. Midwives, so it was declared with a startling lack of evidence, had once been so feared by the male Church that they had been widely persecuted as witches, the ultimate victims in an era of victim feminism.[8] It was argued that domiciliary nurses too had been autonomous practitioners, but their reputation was blackened while hospital nurses, with reasons to be 'grateful and deferential', came under the thumb of domineering doctors and inculcated into proper lower-class subservience.[9] The old-style nurses had found their defenders: not Sarah Gamps at all, but misunderstood victims of history.[10]

Both the traditional and revisionist narratives of nursing history occasionally mentioned the role of nursing sisterhoods, but it was all too obvious that modern nursing was a secular activity. Recent nursing historians have done much to rescue the 'nursing nun' from obscurity.[11] However, the assumption had long been that religious sisterhoods had little 'practical effect' on the development of modern

---

[5]    C. Davies, 'Introduction', in Celia Davies (ed.), *Rewriting Nursing History* (London, 1980), p. 11.

[6]    See, for example, R. Dingwall, A.M. Rafferty and C. Webster, *An Introduction to the Social History of Nursing* (London, 1988).

[7]    S. Hawkins, *Nursing and Women's Labour in the Nineteenth Century* (London, 2010).

[8]    B. Ehrenreich and D. English, *Witches, Midwives, and Nurses* (2nd edn, New York, 1973).

[9]    A. Summers, *Female Lives, Moral States* (Newbury, Berks., 2000), p. 110. Note that this book is a collection of previously published articles, and so reflects concerns of earlier decades.

[10]   See, for example, A.M. Rafferty, *The Politics of Nursing Knowledge* (London, 1996), p. 11.

[11]   See, for example, S. Nelson, *Say Little, Do Much: Nurses, Nuns and Hospitals in the Nineteenth Century* (Philadelphia, PA, 2001).

nursing other than to bequeath its sense of vocation and to reinforce hierarchical power.[12]

In this book we go beyond traditional and revisionist interpretations of the older 'pre-Nightingale' nurses. Instead, we look at these nurses in the context of the pre-industrial nature of the early nineteenth-century workforce and the rough realities of that society. We examine carefully their work environment and living conditions. Our sources reveal that in the early nineteenth century, hospital reformers had good reason to be concerned about the impact of chaotic, inadequate nursing on patient outcomes. Medicine was rapidly changing and gradually becoming more effective – not just because of much-heralded technical advances, but, we argue, a fundamental change in therapeutics. Order, regularity, punctuality, sobriety and industriousness were all middle-class values, but they were also necessary if nurses were to deliver the new health care efficiently. Sarah Gamp's uncertain work ethic was based on contemporary reality – a feature which made Dickens such a powerful force for reform. Hospital nurses were being charged with important aspects of patient care, and although they lacked any voice in hospital governance and frequently worked under appalling conditions, they had become essential pillars of the new hospital medicine. Change in nursing ultimately occurred not because of social factors, but primarily because of the clinical needs of an increasingly effective medical practice.

We examine the evidence, asking fundamental questions such as: 'Who were the hospital nurses?' and 'Were the "winners" in history – secular Nightingale-style trained nurses – always seen as the best way forward for nursing reform?' We distinguish between the different levels of nurses and ask: 'Was it possible for women working under such conditions, with few expectations of training, to even approximate our ideas of effective, compassionate nurses? Were they even expected to be nurses in the modern sense?' Most of all, we look at the ideas held by middle-class Victorians themselves, particularly their assumption that there was no morality without religion. Were the Anglican nursing sisterhoods, now barely recognized as having ever existed, the progenitors of modern nursing? It is time to get off the roller-coaster of competing assumptions and examine what life was like for nurses during the nineteenth century, and how and why so many reformers, great and small, tried to find better, more effective ways to provide hospital nursing. We examine how nursing reform culminated in, rather than began with, the Nightingale system of nursing as practised at St Thomas' Hospital.

In this book we focus on the dominant paradigm of nursing and what caused it to change. Mick Carpenter rightly castigated nursing historians for assuming that 'nursing' refers to general hospital nursing, rather than its many variants, such as psychiatric nursing.[13] We do define nursing as general hospital nursing, but only

---

[12]   For example, Dingwall et al., *An Introduction to the Social History of Nursing*, p. 29.

[13]   M. Carpenter, 'Asylum Nursing before 1914', in Davies, *Rewriting Nursing History*, p. 124.

because it was there that the huge changes in nursing education and practice were first felt. We also focus almost exclusively on the 12 London teaching hospitals. Again, the reason is that the changes in nursing education and practice first occurred in those hospitals. There were numerous renowned hospitals elsewhere in Great Britain, but they looked to the London teaching hospitals for leadership in nursing reform.[14]

A final point to make is about the title. As the date range indicates, this book is not just about nursing before the birth of Florence Nightingale, or even before the Nightingale School of Nursing was founded. Rather, it looks at nursing before the Nightingale model became supreme in the twentieth century, and rather than assume its inevitability, questions why it became the dominant model. Our book continues to 1899 because this was when the last of the Anglican Sisterhoods left the London teaching hospitals. It was the Anglican Sisters, we demonstrate, who were the leaders of nursing reform for much of the nineteenth century.

---

[14]    For example, MRI, WB, 21, 5 December 1864, LGI, WB/3/13, 4 February 1870, WB/3/15, 2 April 1880, and BGH/WB, 21 October 1859. See also S. Wildman, 'Local Nursing Associations in an Age of Nursing Reform: England 1862–1900', *International Perspectives in the History of Nursing Conference*, Royal Holloway College, Windsor, UK, 14–16 September 2010, and S. Wildman, 'Nursing and the Issue of Party in the Church of England: The Case of the Lichfield Diocesan Nursing Association', *Nursing Inquiry*, 16/2 (2009): pp. 94–102.

# Acknowledgements

We would like to thank fellow historians, and especially Trevor Lloyd, Sioban Nelson, Sue Hawkins, Michael Roberts and Janet Likeman. We are very grateful to the many helpful archivists from the archives listed in our bibliography, and to Aleksandra Nikolic, Fisher Library, University of Sydney. Carol Helmstadter, as head, and Judith Godden, as a member, of the nursing team which for more than five years collected material for the nursing volumes in the Collected Works of Florence Nightingale project, would like to thank all those who helped them collect material for the project: this material has proved useful in placing the earlier reforms in context.

Carol thanks the Associated Medical Services and Nancy's Own Foundation as well as many smaller donors for generous funding which helped pay for research in England using the Nightingale papers. Carol also acknowledges with gratitude the Social Science and Humanities Research Council of Canada grant which enabled her to start the research for this book. Judith Godden thanks the School of Public Health, and most recently, the Department of History, where she is an honorary associate, both at the University of Sydney, for their support for her part in the research.

Our greatest debt is to our families, especially Dick Helmstadter and David Godden, for their consistent support and timely assistance when needed.

# List of Abbreviations

**Archives**

| | |
|---|---|
| ASA | All Saints Sisters Archives, Oxford |
| BA | Bermondsey Annals, Convent of Mercy, London |
| BGH | Birmingham General Hospital |
| BL | British Library Additional Manuscripts |
| BUNA | Boston University Nursing Archives |
| CCH | Charing Cross Hospital Archives |
| CSSJD | Community of the Sisters of St John the Divine, Birmingham |
| DK | Kaiserswerth Archives |
| FNM | Florence Nightingale Museum |
| KH | King's College Hospital Archives |
| LGI | Leeds General Infirmary |
| LH | London Hospital Archives |
| LMA | London Metropolitan Archives |
| LPA | Lambeth Palace Archives |
| MRI | Manchester Royal Infirmary |
| NC | Nightingale Collection |
| PHA | Pusey House Archives, Oxford |
| RFH | Royal Free Hospital Archives |
| SBH | St Bartholomew's Hospital |
| SGH | St George's Hospital Archives |
| UCH | University College Hospital |
| WI | Wellcome Institute |

**Other Abbreviations**

| | |
|---|---|
| *BMJ* | *British Medical Journal* |
| BNA | British Nursing Association |
| MBG | Minutes of Board of Governors |
| MHC | Minutes of House Committee |
| *PP* | *Parliamentary Papers* |
| WB | Weekly Board |

# Glossary

**Hospital Administrative Structure**

*House Committee*: The boards of each of the 12 London teaching hospitals delegated the authority to run the day-to-day affairs of the hospital to a small committee of governors. The names for this committee varied from hospital to hospital. It was sometimes called the *Weekly Board* because it met once a week, and sometimes the *Taking In Committee*, stemming from its original function of admitting, or taking in, and discharging patients once a week. At Guy's it was called the *Committee of Committees*, at King's College Hospital the *Committee of Management*, and at University College Hospital the *General Committee*. Despite the different names, these committees performed the same function. The matron reported to the House Committee, except at St Bartholomew's, where she reported to the Treasurer's and Almoners' Committee.

*Servant*: The matron, sisters, doctors and administrative staff were hospital officers. The porters, surgery man, kitchen staff and nurses were hospital servants. In the nineteenth century, 'servant' did not always carry the same meaning as today. For example, the men who governed millions of people in India were called civil servants.

*Steward*: The steward was more or less the equivalent of the matron for the male patients, responsible for maintaining order and discipline among them. He also ordered food and supplies and supervised maintenance of the building. When Dr Steele was hired as medical superintendent at Guy's Hospital, it was the steward's job which he took over.

*Surgery Man*: This hospital servant was essentially a cleaner who worked in the operating theatre, and usually the dead house.

*Treasurer*: In the endowed hospitals, the Treasurer, one of the volunteer board members, was roughly the equivalent of the CEO of a modern hospital. He was unpaid, but was usually given a house and servant.

**Nursing Titles**

These are very confusing because the same word meant different things in different hospitals.

*Assistant nurse*: These were the ordinary nurses. They had different titles in different hospitals. At St Thomas' they were usually called *nurses*, as opposed to the sisters or head nurses. They could also be called *under-nurses* because they worked under the sister. At St Mary's Hospital they were called *diet nurses* because so much of the assistant nurse's time was spent carrying the diet trays up from the kitchen to the wards.

*Extra nurse*: These nurses were what are now called casual nurses, women who could be called on occasionally to work either with individual acute cases or simply as additional help when the wards were especially busy.

*Head nurse*: In the first part of the nineteenth century, this term meant a nurse who was in charge of one or more assistant nurses. In the second half of the century, after training came in, the term acquired a second meaning. 'Head nurse' could mean a trained nurse who was placed in charge of the ward when the sister was either off duty, at lunch or away. The head nurse had become more or less the equivalent of the modern charge nurse.

*Lady*: This term had various meanings. It commonly indicated a woman of the upper classes who did not need to work for a living, and who had personal authority, including the ability to give orders calmly and efficiently.

*Lady Superintendent*: When ladies first entered nursing, they took the title 'lady superintendent' to distinguish themselves from the old lower-middle-class matrons. The new title also indicated that they were responsible for nursing care for which the old matrons bore no responsibility.

*Mrs and Miss*: The Victorians used the title 'Mrs' as a way of showing respect, and not just an indication of marital status. The title 'Miss' almost always indicated that the individual was a single lady. Working-class women were usually referred to simply by their last name with no title. During the Crimean War, Nightingale was an exception in calling the working-class nurses 'Mrs'. For example, she referred to Eliza Roberts, who was unmarried, as 'Mrs Roberts'.

*Night watcher*: These were women who originally, as the title suggests, were hired to come in and watch the patients at night. Traditionally, they lived outside the hospital.

*Nurse*: In some hospitals such as the London and St George's, 'nurse', frequently capitalized, indicated a head nurse as opposed to an assistant or under-nurse. At St George's, Nurses were also called head nurses. In other hospitals, such as the Westminster and the Middlesex, there was only one category of day nurse, and she was called simply 'the nurse'.

*Sister*: This term is especially confusing because it had two meanings. The two medieval hospitals, St Thomas' and St Bartholomew's, had originally been nursed by religious orders, and kept the title 'sister' for their nurses after the Reformation. Guy's was originally founded as an adjunct to St Thomas', and therefore also used the title 'sister'. As the sister in these hospitals was assigned assistant nurses, 'sister' came to mean what other hospitals called a head nurse or Nurse. These women were not religious Sisters as their medieval forebears had been. When the Anglican Sisters entered the field, they were real religious Sisters, women who belonged to a religious order but were also sisters in the sense of head nurses. Adding to the confusion, Elizabeth Fry's nurses were called sisters when they were neither members of a religious order nor head nurses. Later in the century, when St Thomas' nursing gained leadership in the field, the other teaching hospitals began calling their head nurses sisters.

For purposes of clarification, we have capitalized 'sister' when it refers to religious Sisters, and left sister in lower case when it refers to head nurses who did not belong to a religious order.

**Medical Terms**

*Antisepsis*: This is aimed at killing or preventing the growth of germs. In the operating room, antisepsis was most famously provided by Lister's carbolic spray.

*Asepsis*: In contrast to antisepsis, asepsis attempts to create a germ-free environment, or in modern terms, an absence of disease-producing micro-organisms. In the 1890s, aseptic technique involved sterilizing all instruments and dressings. In the first decade of the nineteenth century, sterile gowns, caps, gloves and masks began to be used in the operating room.

*Dresser*: Dressers were medical students whom the senior surgeons selected as their apprentices or helpers. Clinical clerks were the equivalent for physicians.

*Physician's Assistant*: This medical officer was roughly equivalent to a hospital resident today, a person who had just finished medical school and then worked in the hospital to gain a further qualification.

# Chapter 1

# The New Medicine
# and its Dependence on Good Nursing

'One of the greatest difficulties which occur in completing the arrangements of an hospital', young Dr Benjamin Golding wrote in 1819, 'is the procuring of proper persons to act as nurses.'[1] He was far from alone in his opinion; few people in early nineteenth-century London were satisfied with the standard of hospital nursing. Respectable women or 'proper persons' were not interested in hospital nursing because it was considered a menial job, consisting mainly of housework and cleaning up after the patients. Indeed, when investigating the hospital, the Charity Commissioners[2] lumped the patients, furniture and floors together. They described the nurses' work as 'all the usual duties of servants, in waiting on and cleaning the patients, the beds, furniture, wards and stairs',[3] a good illustration of the way the upper classes thought of the lower classes in this age of extreme class-consciousness.

Golding represented the new view of nurses. In 1819 he had recently qualified as a doctor at St Thomas' Hospital and knew that 'as much perhaps depends upon the humane endeavours of a kind and attentive female as upon the ability of the medical attendant'. In many instances good nursing care was all that a doctor could prescribe. Patients could die through a nurse's mismanagement, while there were also, Golding wrote, many instances where it was not medical attention but the 'good nursing and care to administer solace and comfort' which resulted in a patient's recovery.

Over the course of the nineteenth century a series of nursing reforms in the 12 London teaching hospitals produced the 'proper' or respectable nurse whom Golding's generation found in such short supply. In 1819 there was no such thing as a nursing school, and only four of the seven voluntary hospitals then in existence had medical schools – St Bartholomew's, the United Hospitals of St Thomas' and Guy's, and the London. By the end of the century there were 12 London hospitals with medical schools, and each had its own nursing school as well. Established

---

[1]   B. Golding, *An Historical Account of the Origin and Progress of St Thomas's Hospital Southwark* (London, 1819), pp. 214–15. In the nineteenth century, St Thomas' was generally spelled St Thomas's; we use the modern spelling.

[2]   The Charity Commission was a body the government established in 1818 to prevent the abuse of charities and see that their money was correctly and efficiently used. R. Tompson, *The Charity Commission and the Age of Reform* (Toronto, 1979), pp. 99, 159–77.

[3]   LMA/H09/GY/A71, p. 54.

by different groups at different times, each had its own traditions and its own constitution; hence the development of the new nursing services differed from hospital to hospital. However, by the end of the century the so-called 'Nightingale nurse', a respectable and proper person, had emerged as the standard model throughout the English-speaking world.

## The 12 London Teaching Hospitals and their New Mission

Changes in medical practice in the London teaching hospitals forced the development of this new model. 'British medicine changed radically in the seventy years or so that preceded the middle of the nineteenth century,' Roger French and Andrew Wear wrote; 'This was the Age of Reform, in medicine as in politics.'[4] Medical education became increasingly based on science[5] as the learned, classical medicine of the university gave way to a more practical, hands-on training. Medical teaching began to take root in hospitals, and by 1780 the London hospitals were becoming a centre for medical education which rivalled Paris. Medical students walked the wards, some were assigned patient care responsibilities, and all, of course, could observe the old nurses at work and the inability of many to cope with the new regime which the medical schools were introducing. The desperate needs of the Revolutionary and Napoleonic Wars during 1793–1815 required more practically trained doctors, and as historian Susan Lawrence indicated, had a more important impact on medical reform than did later, better-known vocal critics of the medical élite.[6] By 1830 in England, the less formal hospital school had replaced the university as the primary provider of medical education.[7]

The first two of the London teaching hospitals were monastic foundations, St Bartholomew's founded in 1123, and St Thomas' about 1207. Throughout the Middle Ages they were essentially Church-run social service agencies, providing asylum for people who could not support themselves – the lame, the blind, beggars,

---

[4]   R. French and A. Wear (eds), *British Medicine in an Age of Reform* (London, 1991), p. 1.

[5]   R. Porter and W.F. Bynum, 'The Art and Science of Medicine', in W.F. Bynum and R. Porter (eds), *Companion Encyclopedia of the History of Medicine* (2 vols, New York, 1993), vol. 1, p. 7.

[6]   T.N. Bonner, *Becoming a Physician: Medical Education in Britain, France, Germany and the United States 1750–1945* (New York, 1995), pp. 6–8, 14, 31–2, 39, 61–2, 98–9; C. Lawrence, *Medicine in the Making of Modern Britain* (London, 1993), pp. 22–5; S.C. Lawrence, *Charitable Knowledge: Pupils and Practitioners in Eighteenth Century London* (Cambridge, 1996), pp. 91–106; L. Rosner, 'The Growth of Medical Education and the Medical Profession', in I. Loudon (ed.), *Western Medicine: An Illustrated History* (Oxford, 1997), p. 151.

[7]   Lawrence, *Charitable Knowledge*, pp. 162–5; Bonner, *Becoming a Physician*, p. 140.

the chronic sick and the mad, as well as some individuals who were acutely ill and needed medical attention.[8] In the eighteenth century, philanthropists, among whom doctors figured prominently, founded five new hospitals, the Westminster, Guy's, St George's, the London and the Middlesex, to relieve sick, needy and other distressed persons. Their mission was also moral, but incorporated a more medical aim, for it was hoped that medical care would enable the patients to return to active, useful lives. In the nineteenth century, five more hospitals were established: the Royal Free[9] and University College in 1828,[10] Charing Cross in 1834,[11] King's College in 1839 and St Mary's in 1845.

In the older hospitals, the medical schools developed gradually; there were students and lectures for many years before a formal school was established.[12] The first of the formal schools was at Guy's and St Thomas', founded in 1769 and known as the United Hospitals School until 1825, when the two hospitals established separate medical schools. The London formally began its school in 1785, and St Bartholomew's in 1787. St Bartholomew's became more widely known in the medical world simply as 'Bart's'. All the other hospitals started their medical schools between 1821 and 1845. The last four nineteenth-century hospitals to be established, University College, Charing Cross, King's College and St Mary's, were specifically founded to provide clinical practice for medical students as well as for care of the sick poor. Thus medical schools added medical science and research to the hospitals' traditional humanitarian and religious aims.[13]

These 12 public hospitals were all voluntary or charitable foundations: they received no money from the state. St Bartholomew's, St Thomas' and Guy's had large endowments, and were hence often referred to as 'the endowed hospitals', but the other nine hospitals relied principally on current subscriptions and donations to finance their operating costs, a fact which was to have a major impact on the development of the new nursing, for it had to compete with medical schools and building programmes for scarce resources.[14]

---

[8]   B. Abel-Smith, *The Hospitals 1800–1948: A Study in Social Administration in England and Wales* (London, 1964), pp. 10–11, 14–15.

[9]   Founded as the London General Institution for the Gratuitous Cure of Malignant Diseases, it became the Free Hospital in 1835, and was granted the title Royal in 1837.

[10]   Founded as the University Dispensary, it was replaced in 1834 by the North London Hospital. In 1837 it changed its name to University College Hospital, though it was often called by its previous title throughout the nineteenth century.

[11]   Founded in 1818 as the West London Infirmary and Dispensary.

[12]   W.F. Bynum, *Science and the Practice of Medicine in the Nineteenth Century* (Cambridge, 1994), pp. 48–9.

[13]   Bonner, *Becoming a Physician*, pp. 50–52; Lawrence, *Charitable Knowledge*, pp. 336–8.

[14]   Abel-Smith, *The Hospitals*, pp. 4–5.

4 NURSING BEFORE NIGHTINGALE, 1815–1899

## The New Demands on Hospital Nurses

The new 'scientific' hospital medicine with its focus on medical care rather than social service forced radical changes in nursing.[15] The emphasis on supportive therapeutics placed far greater responsibility on the nurses and made the shortcomings of the old nurses painfully obvious. In simplest terms, the old therapeutics tried to restore a balance in the patient's physiology. Treatments consisted of 'elevating' or 'stimulating' a weak patient, usually with alcohol and a generous diet, and 'depleting' or 'lowering' a feverish or overexcited patient with purgatives, emetics, blisters, low diets and bleeding. Most disease conditions had traditionally been thought to require lowering,[16] but the new medicine favoured supportive treatments.

As well as the change in therapeutics, doctors were conceiving disease in a different way. Historically, disease was identified with sin, or a visitation from God to improve the moral character of the sick person. Henry Wentworth Acland (later Sir Henry, and Regius Professor of Medicine at Oxford) entered St George's Hospital as a medical student in 1840. He explained his understanding of disease at the time:

> He knew of disease only that it was from God; that it was a remedy applied to
> the body to cure the disorders of a sinning soul; a mark of chastisement; an act
> of love from the hand of a wise Father.[17]

When the Anglicans declared in their General Confession, 'We have left undone those things which we ought to have done, and done those things which we ought not to have done, and there is no health in us,' they were referring to their physical health equally as much as their spiritual health. The two could not be separated: in the eighteenth century, health and virtue were ideally one.[18]

This holistic view of health is exemplified by the use of corporal punishment as a part of medical treatment. In 1819, venereal disease patients, especially women patients at St Thomas', were often privately whipped and then admonished to pursue a better life before they were discharged. The hospital had removed the public whipping post and stocks only a few years previously.[19] The new scientific doctors were challenging the moral origins of disease, placing its causes on a more

15 Dingwall et al., *An Introduction to the Social History of Nursing*, p. 23.

16 J.H. Warner, *The Therapeutic Perspective: Medical Practice, Knowledge, and Identity in America 1820–1885* (Cambridge, 1986), pp. 85–6, 91–6; I.A. Burney, 'Medicine in the Age of Reform', in A. Burns and J. Innes (eds), *Rethinking the Age of Reform: Britain 1780–1850* (Cambridge, 2003), p. 167; Lawrence, *Medicine in the Making*, pp. 9–12.

17 J.B. Atlay, *Sir Henry Wentworth Acland, Regius Professor of Medicine in the University of Oxford: A Memoir* (London, 1903), p. 90.

18 Lawrence, *Medicine in the Making*, pp. 62–3.

19 Golding, *An Historical Account*, pp. 220–21.

anatomical basis, but throughout the nineteenth century sickness remained loaded with moral and religious meaning.[20] Ideally, in order to create the right healing environment, the nurses had to be morally respectable.[21] This view did not change throughout the century, but the new emphasis on anatomy meant nurses now had to have some knowledge of anatomy and physiology.

As the new medicine took hold in the teaching hospitals, it gradually transformed them into curative institutions. Traditionally, doctors were allowed to admit emergencies themselves, but the Taking-In or House Committee admitted most patients on the recommendation of a governor. Many of these patients needed only periods of rest, but the doctors sought a different type of patient – acutely ill persons as well as emergencies, patients whom they could help and who were useful for their teaching. The tension between the doctors and the governors at the London on this issue was typical. In 1822 the governors told the medical staff they had no right to admit patients unless they were accident victims.[22] Doctors were admitting patients who were not always urgent or accident cases every day of the week, when only the House Committee had the right to admit patients, and then only once a week on Tuesday at 1 p.m. The doctors admitted so many patients that there were frequently no beds available for the persons whom the governors referred.[23] This had a financial implication because governors were less inclined to donate money when the people they recommended as patients were turned away. The increase in acute cases meant a much heavier workload for the nurses, with exponentially increased responsibility for the many more severely ill patients whom the doctors were admitting.

Furthermore, new ideas about hygiene, the spread of infection, the treatment of pain, new and more daring operations, and finally, the heavy feeding schedules which the new supportive treatments required all demanded more skilled nursing. In the jails, ships of the Royal Navy and the overcrowded towns, the new clinical doctors met epidemic and endemic fevers. Treating diseases of populations forced them to rethink two concepts of eighteenth-century medicine: first, that each case was unique, and second, that disease itself was an individual, localized entity. While some considered poverty the root cause of fevers, others began thinking of dirt, indolence and moral laxity as the source. There developed a new stress on dirt, which was associated with disorder, while cleanliness came to be identified with order, morality and discipline, in no place better illustrated than in the Royal Navy. Cleanliness was also a sign of civilized gentility. The 'great unwashed', the

---

[20]     Lawrence, *Medicine in the Making*, pp. 62–3.

[21]     C.E. Rosenberg, 'Florence Nightingale on Contagion', in Charles E. Rosenberg (ed.), *Healing and History: Essays for George Rosen* (New York, 1979), pp. 124–7.

[22]     LH/A4/19, 17 and 31 December 1822, 7 and 14 January 1823; see also LMA/H02/WH/A1/28, 31 October 1827.

[23]     LH/A17/5, 17 April 1827.

poor, became objects of the new hygiene as well as of stigmatization.[24] The new concern with cleanliness greatly increased the drudgery of hospital nurses, for they were responsible for the state of cleanliness of the hospital as well as that of the patients.

The old medicine had considered infection unavoidable, and even necessary for healing. Wounds were therefore often deliberately kept open so that what was believed to be the healing 'laudable' pus could form and drain. Foreign bodies such as strips of thread or pea beans were often introduced into wounds to prevent them from healing quickly and cleanly. From the end of the eighteenth century, however, English surgeons increasingly tried to promote healing by first intention – that is, the two sides of the wound reuniting quickly without forming granulation tissue. By the 1840s many of these surgeons believed that using single sponges and dressings on multiple patients, and even their own hands and instruments, spread infection.[25] In 1854, a good decade before Lister's publications, Florence Nightingale was not unusual in thinking that using the same sponge on the wounds of many different soldiers, as was then being done in Scutari, spread 'Fever, Cholera, Gangrene, Lice, Bugs, Fleas & may be Erysipelas'.[26]

By the early 1860s, when the physician John Bristowe of St Thomas' and surgeon Timothy Holmes of St George's made their study of the hospitals of the United Kingdom, they reported 'remarkable changes' had occurred since the beginning of the century in the treatment of many forms of disease, especially fevers and other acute illnesses. 'Depletion has fallen into disuse, and has been replaced by a nourishing and stimulating plan of treatment,' they wrote. Stimulants were administered freely, while bleeding, emetics and mercury, although still used, were used 'rarely and with extreme caution'. Bristowe and Holmes reported that a clean technique in the local treatment of wounds was becoming standard. Throwing dressings away after one use was becoming more common, while even in hospitals where sponges were still used, the sponge was assigned to a specific patient and subsequently destroyed or chemically purified.[27] As with the cleanliness of the wards, it was the nurses who had to supply the clean sponges, clean instruments and make the disposable dressings – a far more time-consuming task than washing used dressings and providing the one basin of water and sponge with which the old surgeons went down the ward from patient to patient.

In the 1830s and 1840s, well before anaesthesia and antisepsis came in, surgeons were making rapid and unprecedented advances in anatomical and physiological

---

[24]   Lawrence, *Medicine in the Making*, pp. 22–5; A. Wear, 'The History of Personal Hygiene', in Bynum and Porter (eds), *Companion Encyclopedia*, vol. 2, pp. 1,301–5.

[25]   P. Stanley, *For Fear of Pain: British Surgery 1790–1850* (New York, 2003), pp. 147–51.

[26]   BL 43393, fol. 14. Erysipelas is a local febrile disease causing inflammation of the skin, often called St Anthony's Fire. It was one of the four classical nineteenth-century hospital diseases.

[27]   *PP*, 1864 vol. 28, pp. 483–85; see also BGH/WB, 5 December 1862.

knowledge. They were performing new and daring operations, many of which kept the fully conscious patient on the table for protracted lengths of time – tying off aneurysms,[28] operations on fused joints and excision of diseased bones and joints. This new surgery was called 'conservative' because rather than amputating, it conserved limbs by excising diseased tissue.[29] More operations, with what was then a high risk of post-operative haemorrhage, required skilled nursing around the clock. Some surgeons even said that post-operative nursing care was more important in determining the outcome than surgical skill.[30] With the introduction of anaesthesia in the late 1840s, post-anaesthetic care was added to the already greatly expanded duties of the surgical nurses.

From the 1750s, as part of the broader humanitarian movement, a new view emerged of pain as unnecessary, cruel and something to be avoided. One example of this belief is the anti-vivisection movement which was mobilized so effectively in the 1820s. By the 1830s doctors were adopting the view that pain, rather than being a stimulant, exacerbated the effects of shock and further weakened an already enfeebled patient. Previously, it had been thought that pain helped sustain vitality during surgery. When in 1854 Sir John Hall warned his medical officers in the Crimea against using chloroform for amputation cases when the soldier was in a state of shock, he explained that 'the smart of the knife is a powerful stimulant'. He was not being sadistic, but simply reflecting the older view that it was better 'to hear a man bawl lustily than to see him sink silently into the grave' as a result of loss of consciousness. Opium became a mainstay of therapeutics for chronic diseases and to ease the pain of the dying. Pain relief became a major function of the doctor,[31] but in the hospitals it was the nurses, not the doctors, who administered the analgesics – another addition to their growing number of duties.

Of all the additional burdens which the new medicine placed on the nurses, perhaps the most time-consuming was the emphasis on generous, nourishing diets and the frequent feeding which they required. The nursing care of Henry Franklin illustrates these new demands. He was admitted to King's College Hospital in November 1849 with tetanus, from which he died two days later. He was treated first with fomentations[32] to the jaws and throat, and because he had lockjaw and could not swallow, beef tea enemas throughout the day, plus an enema of starch

---

[28]   A dilatation of an artery which is very likely to burst, producing major haemorrhage with fatal consequences.

[29]   C. Lawrence, 'Democratic, Divine and Heroic: The History and Historiography of Surgery', in C. Lawrence (ed.), *Medical Theory, Surgical Practice: Studies in the History of Surgery* (New York, 1992), pp. 24–5; Stanley, *For Fear of Pain*, pp. 67–9.

[30]   Ibid., pp. 49–52, 144, 146–7.

[31]   S. Snow, *Operations without Pain: The Practice and Science of Anesthesia in Victorian Britain* (London, 2006), pp. 21–4, 28, 99, 142–5; Stanley, *For Fear of Pain*, p. 305.

[32]   Fomentations were flannels, soaked in hot water which was frequently medicated, and applied to the skin or a wound to relieve pain.

and opium at night. The next day, as well as the beef tea enemas, he had a tobacco fomentation and a quinine enema,[33] together with frequent inhalations of chloroform and air to relax his muscles.[34] While a medical student or the physician himself normally administered chloroform, making and administering the fomentations and enemas was the nurse's job. One can imagine how much time Franklin's treatments took, as they entailed regular application of two different fomentations and three types of enemas. At the same time, Franklin's nurse was responsible for cleaning the ward and for 14 other patients.

As a result of all these changes during the first half of the nineteenth century, hospital medicine became increasingly dependent on skilled, conscientious nursing care. But as Golding pointed out, it was extremely difficult to find proper persons who could be relied on to implement medical orders.

## Hospital Nurses as Domestic Servants

'Proper' nurses were scarce in part because hospital nursing staffs were not designed to meet the needs of the new medicine. In the early nineteenth century nurses were primarily maids-of-all-work whose principal job was cleaning, not patient care. There were three classes of nurse under the direction of a matron: the sisters, sometimes called head nurses or (usually capitalized) Nurse, the assistant or ordinary day nurses, and the night watch or night nurses. The matron was a paid hospital officer, but was subordinate to the other hospital officers. Golding described her as superintending 'those departments which could not be so well regulated by a person of the other sex',[35] a reflection of the contemporary ideal of society divided by gender into women's and men's spheres. She was not a nurse, but rather a housekeeper in charge of the kitchen maids as well. She came from a somewhat higher social class than the nurses, for she had to be able to read and write. She was responsible for the inventory, the cleanliness and good order of the hospital, and the proper behaviour of her staff. Nursing care was not her responsibility.

At the beginning of the nineteenth century much of the sisters' work remained cleaning and washing. St Thomas' regulations were typical. The sisters were to keep the ward constantly neat and clean, to carry out all the filth, to wash or cause to be washed all the weak patients' clothes, to give medicines as directed, and to clean half the ward. In addition, the sister was responsible for having some sober patient offer the blessing at each meal and for maintaining order among the patients. The sister had an assistant nurse, and if she was sick or did not appear for work, the sister applied to the matron for a replacement.[36]

---

[33]   Quinine was then considered a stimulant.

[34]   R.B. Todd, *Clinical Lectures on Paralysis, Certain Diseases of the Brain and Other Affections of the Nervous System* (2nd edn, London, 1856), pp. 406–13, 423–4.

[35]   Abel-Smith, *The Hospitals*, pp. 7–8; Golding, *An Historical Account*, pp. 189–215.

[36]   LMA/H01/ST/A25; LMA/H09/GY/A71, pp. 673–74, 735–8.

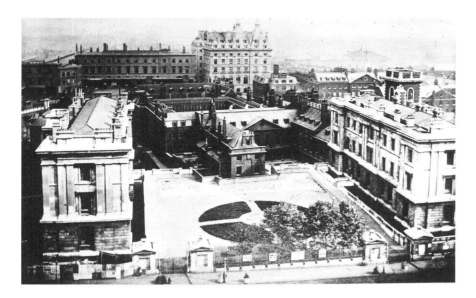

Figure 1.1     St Thomas' Hospital just before it was demolished in 1862. The hospital was built at the end of the seventeenth and beginning of the eighteenth centuries on a plan of four enclosed squares. The central kitchen was in the second square. The assistant nurses had to carry the meal trays to the wards in the other squares in all kinds of weather. Because this took so much of their time, the assistant nurses were sometimes called diet nurses.

*Source*: By kind permission of the Trustees of the Guy's and St Thomas' Charity, London.

The assistant nurses attended the surgeons when they dressed the patients, taking away the used bandages, bolsters and rags and providing clean ones. They gave the enemas and vomits, prepared the water gruels and pottage for the weak patients, cleaned the other half of the ward, and scoured the beds, floors, tables, benches, passages, stairs, garrets, beer cans, broth pails and plates. With the assistance of convalescent patients, they carried the meals from the kitchen to the wards and helped the butler to distribute the beer and see that the patients helping them did not drink it. Finally, they cleaned the incontinent patients and their bedding.[37]

In 1819 Golding referred to nurses as 'female domestics', and used the term 'menial' interchangeably with 'nurse'.[38] Thirty-eight years later, John Flint South, a senior surgeon at St Thomas', thought 'ward servants' would be a better name for the women whom St Thomas' called 'nurses' or 'assistant nurses'.[39] Few

---

[37]  LMA/H01/ST/A25.

[38]  Golding, *An Historical Account*, p. 203 and passim.

[39]  J.F. South, *Facts Relating to Hospital Nurses* (London, 1857), p. 9.

would have argued with these two doctors. In the eighteenth and earlier nineteenth centuries, nurses were thought of as domestic servants, not health care workers. Sick nursing was not listed as a separate occupation in the national census until 1861.[40]

At St Thomas', the third team, the night watchers, lived outside the hospital and came in for a 15-hour shift, starting at 7 p.m. in winter and 8 p.m. in summer. As well as 'watching' the patients, they helped clean the wards, and were to check the patients' condition frequently, and if any seemed to have changed for the worse, to immediately inform the sister.[41] The ability to assess patients, later a hallmark of the new nurses, was not mentioned in the day nurses' duties because it was expected that the sister or the medical officers would do this. For lack of anyone else, this responsibility fell on the night nurses, but no one thought to give them any training in assessment skills and they did not have the opportunity to learn from the more experienced nurses and sisters for they were on duty alone at night. Consequently, they were usually the least competent of the three nursing teams.

What was the labour pool from which hospitals recruited their nurses? Hospital nurses were usually widows, single mothers or women in their late thirties and forties who had failed to maintain themselves in domestic service. Domestic service employed the largest number of women in England, and hospital nursing formed the lowest rung in that hierarchical occupation. Beyond domestic service, street selling, prostitution and the various lower levels of the clothing trade were the only possibilities for unskilled women, and these occupations often provided only irregular employment.[42] 'In England,' Florence Nightingale wrote in 1857, employment opportunities for women were 'few, narrow and overcrowded'. In London and other cities, she said, there were large numbers of prostitutes, and even more women occupied 'a hideous border-land', combining prostitution with other work, including nursing. About an equal number of women, again including nurses, rejected prostitution, and accordingly had to 'struggle through their lives as they can, on precarious work and insufficient wages'.[43] Nurses fell into Nightingale's last two categories of workers.

[40]   P. Williams, 'Religion, Respectability and the Origins of the Modern Nurse', in French and Wear (eds), *British Medicine in an Age of Reform*, pp. 232–3.

[41]   LMA/H01/ST/A25.

[42]   LMA/H01/ST/C2/1 and 2, passim; WI SA/QNI/W4; T. McBride, *The Domestic Revolution: The Modernisation of Household Service in England and France* (London, 1976), p. 101; S. Alexander, *Women's Work in Nineteenth-century London: A Study of the Years 1820–50* (London, 1983), pp. 20–22. See also Sir E. Cook, *The Life of Florence Nightingale* (2 vols, London, 1913), vol. 1, p. 445; M. Goodman, *Experiences of an English Sister of Mercy* (London, 1862), pp. 8–61. Hours and days of work were similar in all the hospitals. See, for example, LH/A1/5.

[43]   Florence Nightingale, 'Introducing Female Nurses into Military Hospitals', in L.R. Seymer (ed.), *Selected Writings of Florence Nightingale* (New York, 1954), p. 6.

Nursing offered one of the few employment opportunities for women who had no training of any kind and either had no money for apprenticeship fees or were too old to be apprenticed. Hospital nurses were essentially cleaning women, but while cleaning women were usually hired by the day, nursing offered steady work – in fact, too steady. In the first part of the century, nurses normally had no days off; they worked seven days a week, 52 weeks of the year. Assistant nurses normally worked a 16- to 17-hour shift, from 6 a.m. till 10 or 11 p.m.[44] If they wanted a day off, they had to find and pay their own substitute.[45] These hours were standard in domestic service for a maid-of-all-work,[46] which is what an assistant nurse equated to, but compared unfavourably to industrial occupations where a 12-hour day six days a week was more usual.[47]

## Hospital Organizational Culture in the First Half of the Nineteenth Century: 'A Total Want of System and Regularity'

A look at the organizational culture of hospitals at the beginning of the nineteenth century indicates how different hospital life was from that of today. Most patients were not seriously ill; many were ambulatory and quite able to roister about the hospital wards and grounds. Since many were permitted to leave the hospital during the day, many found shelter in the welcoming environment of the pubs and frequently returned drunk. They could also then smuggle liquor into the hospital.[48]

Drink was the national vice, a major problem not only among the working classes, but throughout all levels of society. As water was unsafe to drink, all hospitals provided their patients and staff with beer. Furthermore, medical men prescribed alcohol liberally as they believed it strengthened physical stamina. It was not until the 1870s, with the impact of the temperance movement, that the medical profession began to effectively challenge the belief that alcohol was a restorative.[49]

The patients' fondness for alcohol made the porters' job especially difficult. Every hospital had a porter whose major task was preventing the patients and

---

[44]    LH/A1/5.

[45]    See, for example, KH/CM/M2, 21 June 1843.

[46]    P. Horn, *The Rise and Fall of the Victorian Servant* (New York, 1975), pp. 49–51.

[47]    K. Theodore Hoppen, *The Mid-Victorian Generation 1846–86* (Oxford, 1998), p. 81. H.-J. Voth, *Time and Work in England 1750–1830* (Oxford, 2000), pp. 268–270, estimated that between 1760 and 1830, the total number of hours worked increased by approximately 20 per cent, largely because there were fewer days off.

[48]    Abel-Smith, *The Hospitals*, pp. 10–11; Golding, *An Historical Account*, pp. 202, 239–40.

[49]    W. Blizard, *Suggestions for the Improvement of Hospitals and Other Charitable Institutions* (London, 1796), p. 60; B. Harrison, *Drink and the Victorians: The Temperance Question in England 1815–72* (Pittsburgh, PA, 1971), pp. 37–41, 306–9.

hospital staff from going in and out of the hospital without written permission. They were also supposed to prevent patients from smuggling in alcohol and to stop visitors from taking hospital property, such as food, soap and candles, out of the hospital. In addition, the porters were to admit only proper visitors, appropriately dressed. This rule was aimed at preventing prostitutes from plying their trade within the hospital. St Thomas' had four porters, each paid £50 a year – a very good salary for unskilled men – but they were not very effective. Notwithstanding their efforts, and sometimes with their help, patients and their friends continually smuggled provisions out of the hospital and alcohol into it.[50]

Two quite different hospitals provide characteristic illustrations of hospital organizational culture in the early nineteenth century. One, the Westminster Hospital, had less than 100 beds and did not yet have a medical school.[51] The other, the London Hospital, had approximately 250 beds[52] and a medical school founded in the eighteenth century.

## The Westminster Hospital

The Westminster's elderly matron, Mrs Jane Mortteras, had many problems with her staff of four day and four night nurses. In April 1818 the House Surgeon reported Night Nurse Thomason was drunk and failed to give a patient his medicine. She insisted that she had, but the patient said she had not.[53] Failure to carry out doctors' orders was one of the commonest complaints. In June 1817 Mortteras dismissed two nurses for incompetence. As well as drunkenness and incompetence, there were problems with nurses leaving their patients unattended, going in and out of the hospital without permission, extorting money from the patients and ordering extra beer for themselves at hospital expense.[54]

In May 1818 the Chairman of the Board reprimanded Mortteras for 'many instances of gross neglect'. In a lengthy letter of resignation she defended herself while pointing out that, as she was either 77 or 78 years old, she could not expect another appointment. She described how she had been elected matron in 1794 at a salary of £20 a year plus a 3 guinea gratuity.[55] She was never paid the gratuity, but when she discovered that other hospital officers were receiving theirs, she applied for the arrears. She was then convinced to forgo it because the hospital was five quarters behind in paying its bills. Mortteras then shut a small ward and decreased the number of nurses from eight to six, which saved £100 a year. She

---

[50]   Golding, *An Historical Account*, pp. 200–202, 240.

[51]   LMA/H02/WH/A1/31, 29 May 1838.

[52]   A.E. Clark-Kennedy, *The London: A Study in the Voluntary Hospital System* (2 vols, London, 1963), vol. 1, pp. 231–3.

[53]   LMA/H02/WH/A1/25, 22 April 1818.

[54]   Ibid., 17 January, 8 and 29 May 1816, 2 April, 18 June, 1 October 1817, 6 January, 27 October 1819.

[55]   A guinea was £1 1s.

herself took on the job of steward. The steward's salary was £40 annually plus a 10 guinea gratuity and 2 guineas for a messenger, a total of £52 12s. Nevertheless, the governors raised her salary by only £6 (to £26 a year) and she received a £5 gratuity only after presenting a statement of arrears for three years. At the same time some officers had their salaries trebled. As matron, Mortteras was responsible for every article of consumption in the hospital. She felt she had made great savings on beds, furniture and sheets; in addition, she had been a good fundraiser, obtaining benefactions, trustees and subscribers for the hospital.[56] Her only mention of nursing was the dismissal of the two nurses. She obviously considered the nursing, as did most matrons at this time, less important than her other responsibilities of housekeeping, fundraising and saving the hospital money.

The board thought the new matron, Mrs Ann Cox, an improvement, but she also seemed to accept disorder as part of hospital culture. In October 1821 four nurses helped some patients' friends pass porter 'and other improper things' over the garden wall, enabling some patients to get drunk. The board installed new gates, raised the wall three feet higher and put glass bottle capping in the cement on top to prevent further similar occurrences. The following spring, when the governors inspected the hospital they found a Dickensian scene in the cellar. Windows were broken and homeless street urchins were using it as a place to sleep. The boys came in and out daily, leaving it in a shameful state, full of filth and carrion. At the same time, although the porters were supposed to search patients and visitors' baskets and bundles, they were still smuggling large amounts of liquor into the hospital.[57]

The nurses were by no means the only rowdy employees who sometimes left their patients unattended. In 1816 the apothecary and house surgeon complained about the surgery man, saying he was impertinent, neglected his duty and was absent without leave a good deal of the time. The chaplain was also delinquent: he refused to visit the wards unless he was better paid. Claiming that he had sent his lancets away to be sharpened, the house surgeon refused to get out of bed to see a patient with a head injury who needed to be bled.[58] A decade later, Mr Bond, the apothecary and senior resident officer, complained to the House Committee about another house surgeon, Mr Casey. One night Casey and his house pupil and friends held a drunken riotous party. Bond asked the revellers to leave. They refused to go, and when he asked a second time, Casey seized him by the throat and threatened to murder him. Bond managed to get away and summon assistance to evict Casey's friends. Casey was still recuperating in bed two days later when the committee met, so the governors had to wait another week to reprimand him.[59] His conduct was not considered sufficiently outrageous to warrant dismissal.

---

[56]  LMA/H02/WH/A/25, 13 and 27 May 1818.
[57]  LMA/H02/WH/A1/26, 10 and 24 October 1821, 3 April, 26 June, 29 May 1822.
[58]  LMA/H02/WH/A1/25, 7 February, 20 March, 22 May, 3 July, 19 June 1816.
[59]  LMA/H01/WH/A1/27, 10 and 17 May 1826.

When a committee was set up in November 1826 to investigate a porter who was embezzling money from the beer account, it found multiple other problems, the worst in the apothecary's department. He did not appear for work until 11 a.m. or 12 noon, and then spent up to an hour and a half visiting the wards, so he could not dispense his medicines until 1 p.m. Yet the out-patients were told to come at 11 a.m., but often did not get their medicines until after 4 p.m. The in-patients were supposed to get their medicines no later than two hours after they were ordered, but usually got them at 7 p.m., and sometimes not until 9 p.m. The apothecary's shop was left open, and while he was away, the surgery man dispensed dangerous medicines such as digitalis, mercury and opium without labels.

The medical care was unsatisfactory. The house surgeon did not always go into the wards to give the nurses their instructions. The position of house pupil was not an efficient one, but rather a sinecure. The matron seldom made her first visit to the wards before 10 a.m., and only visited them irregularly. Furthermore, she was not always in the kitchen as required when meals were served to see that they were properly prepared. She also hired and even fired servants and nurses without the sanction of the board, whereas she had only the right to suspend them. The nurses did not always carry out the physicians' orders. They frequently admitted patients to the wards with their clothes on without the prescribed bath, with the result that vermin proliferated in the beds. The board's most immediate concern was the way patients and staff went out of the hospital without permission. They reinforced the rule that patients, nurses and servants were never to leave the hospital without signing out. The ad hoc committee summarized their hospital administration as a 'total want of system and regularity in almost every department of the establishment'.[60]

*The London Hospital*

The medical school at the London Hospital added many more complications, and made the failings of the nurses much more obvious and significant. While the other London teaching hospitals were run by committees of volunteer governors, the London had a professional administrator from 1806. John Jenkinson served as apothecary and administrator from 1810 until 1818, followed by the Rev. William Valentine, who held the dual position of administrator and chaplain with the title House Governor.[61] Valentine struggled valiantly for over 20 years to establish a fairer approach to the hospital's working-class employees as well as what the Victorians called better 'moral discipline', or what we now call social order.

There were constant complaints about the nurses. As in all hospitals, they did their personal washing in the wards, a universal practice Jenkinson found very objectionable. He suggested that the wash house should be enlarged so that they could do their washing there. Given that the nurses were supposed to be in their

60   Ibid., 1 and 8 November, 13 and 20 December 1826, 14 March 1827.
61   LH/A17/1, frontispage.

wards from 6 a.m. until 10 or 11 p.m., it is hard to see how they could have legitimately found time to do their washing elsewhere. The arrangements for the nurses' meals were a constant source of trouble. Jenkinson objected to the nurses cooking their meals at the ward fireplace[62] although this was a standard and allowed practice in all the hospitals because there was nowhere else where they could cook. As well, as the governors at the Middlesex pointed out in 1847, 'the very uncertain and variable as well as unpleasant nature' of the nurses' work made it impossible for them to have a fixed hour for dinner.[63]

In 1815 Jenkinson explained that the nurses and other servants of the hospital were frequently accused of stealing money from patients and visitors, but he found this difficult to prove, in part because the patients also stole things. Furthermore, the nurses stole property from helpless patients. 'We must do something to protect the property of the dying, dead and those incapable of doing it for themselves,' he insisted. He suggested the nurses make an inventory of the money and clothes of each patient who was unable to look after his possessions, and give the list to him to keep in his office.[64]

In 1818 Sir William Blizard, senior surgeon at the London and a President of the Royal College of Surgeons, and Drs Buxton and Robertson came as guests to the House Committee. They tried to address the nursing problems, telling the committee they needed a more 'respectable class' of woman to serve as nurses. They did not ask for women with nursing expertise because such expertise was not generally recognized in 1818. They complained of the high rate of turnover among the nurses, and suggested financial rewards for longer service. Nurses should wear a uniform, Blizard and his colleagues said, should never leave the hospital without written permission, and should not do their washing in the wards. To encourage more conformity with the regulations, the governors allotted 80 guineas a year for gratuities for good conduct and longer service.[65]

The gratuities were not very successful. The House Committee continued to report that the nurses, servants and others ignored hospital regulations. Notices stating that servants would be dismissed if they did not follow the rules were placed in conspicuous parts of the hospital;[66] there were already large signs in the wards forbidding patients and visitors to tip the nurses or servants.[67] Servants in large private homes expected tips from visitors in recompense for the extra work they caused,[68] but in the hospitals the nurses did not wait on the visitors.

Medical students added to the general tone of disorder in the hospital. They were young compared with modern students, often starting at age 14, and were

---

[62]  LH/A1/5; LH/A17/2, 30 January 1816.
[63]  MH/MBG, 23 February 1847.
[64]  LH/A17/1, 5 and 26 December 1815.
[65]  LH/A5/16, 19 December 1818.
[66]  LH/A4/9, 12 February 1822.
[67]  LH/A5/16, 28 November 1815.
[68]  McBride, *The Domestic Revolution*, p. 57.

widely considered rowdy, boisterous and lacking in civility. While there were many exceptions, in general their unruly reputation was well founded.[69] The moral disorder, as the Victorians called the want of order, control and authority, extended into the sexual realm. The issue was compounded by the assumption of many upper-class men that working-class women and girls were sexually available.[70] Hospital governors worried about the predatory attitudes of the medical students. These concerns were behind Valentine's complaint in December 1827, when he found two medical students 'making a riotous noise at 8 p.m. Saturday evening, singing, hallooing and leaping'. One of them grabbed a ten-year-old girl and a nurse as he leapt and hallooed his way through the wards, while another, W. Watkins, used abusive language when Valentine asked them to stop. Valentine said Watkins was constantly in the women's wards although he had no patients there.[71]

While the problems with the medical students could be attributed to the grim realities of the dissection room and wards, as well as to youthful over-exuberance and sexuality, Valentine's difficulties with the apothecary were of a different nature. There were constant complaints because this senior resident medical officer did not keep his books properly, went out and got drunk with the medical students, stayed out of the hospital after the 11 p.m. curfew, and then came in, not through the gates where the porter would see him, but through a window, sometimes as late as 3 a.m. He was away from the hospital so much that he could not perform his duties properly. As was common, such misbehaviour did not result in dismissal – on the contrary, in 1829, and despite Valentine's objections, the Board of Governors voted the apothecary a large increase in salary.[72]

Medical training at this time relied heavily on teaching by dissection, making this the age of the anatomists and body-snatchers, or resurrection men. Because the law allowed only those few bodies of convicted criminals to be dissected, there was a huge trade in corpses which were stolen from graveyards. Historically, dissection was the ultimate punishment, reserved for the worst criminals. It made customary funeral observances impossible, and was considered a gross assault on the integrity and identity of the body and upon the repose of the soul. The prospect of being dissected was horrifying to most Christians, for they believed in physical resurrection. Many thought the soul remained in the body until the last trumpet sounded to call the dead from their graves. Dissection left little but the bones for the soul to reside

---

[69] Bonner, *Becoming a Physician*, pp. 74–5; Atlay, *Sir Henry Wentworth Acland*, pp. 81–4; Stanley, *For Fear of Pain*, p. 168.

[70] S. Marcus, *The Other Victorians: A Study of Sexuality and Pornography in Mid-nineteenth-century England* (2nd edn, New York, 1985), pp. 128–60.

[71] LH/A17/5, 4 December 1827.

[72] LH/A17/6, 24 March 1829. One possibility is that the apothecary benefited from the system of patronage; see J.M. Bourne, *Patronage and Society in Nineteenth-century England* (London, 1986).

in, and body parts were often sold separately.[73] In addition, there were anxieties about the ability of medicine to accurately determine death[74] and fears about acts of sexual indecency in the dissection room.[75] As the medical schools expanded in the 1820s, the shortage of corpses became more acute, and before the Anatomy Act of 1832 which allowed unclaimed bodies of those who died in workhouses to be sent to medical schools for dissecting, hospital cemeteries were a magnet for body-snatchers.[76] At the London, with the approval of the House Committee, the surgeons and their pupils paid the porters to disinter bodies in the hospital cemetery for dissection. The governors did so, they said, 'with as much secrecy and delicacy as possible'. They gave the surgeons 'every facility except their public concurrence'.[77]

Jenkinson and Valentine recognized that burying patients in hospital cemeteries and then quickly exhuming them was standard practice in all the teaching hospitals; they could not prevent it, but they tried to minimize its ill effects. Jenkinson noted in 1811 that the London's burying ground was 'more infested with resurrection men than it ought or need to be'. Mock funerals were often held in hospitals for the benefit of the relatives. Valentine refused to read the funeral service over coffins full of stones and seldom permitted a patient to be dissected before burial.[78] When in November 1822 one of the assistant nurses died in the hospital, the surgeons did not dissect her corpse, but they opened her head and body without her husband's permission, causing great distress among the hospital servants. Valentine objected strongly. 'If the same reasonable and proper attention to the feelings of the friends and servants dying in the hospital is not to be observed,' he protested, 'another very great obstacle will be thrown in the way of obtaining respectable persons for the situations in the house.'[79]

In August 1823, body-snatchers tried to steal a body which had been buried the previous day. The patients heard them and shouted out of the windows,

---

[73] R. Richardson, *Death, Dissection and the Destitute* (London, 1987), pp. 76–7; J.M.T. Ford (ed.), *A Medical Student at St Thomas's Hospital 1801–1802: The Weekes Family Letters* (London, 1987), pp. 56, 63, 93, 131, 138.

[74] H. MacDonald, *Human Remains: Episodes in Human Dissection* (Carlton, Victoria, 2005), p. 12.

[75] A. Bashford, *Purity and Pollution: Gender, Embodiment and Victorian Medicine* (London, 1998), pp. 113–22.

[76] MacDonald, *Human Remains*, p.12; H. MacDonald, *Possessing the Dead* (Carlton, Victoria, 2010), pp. 12, 216, demonstrates that the main impact of the Anatomy Act was to replace grave robbing with dissection without consent of the unburied dead in mortuaries of hospitals and other institutions, to the continuing distress of friends and relatives. Such practices did much to reinforce popular prejudice against hospitals and their staff.

[77] LH/A17/3, 2 September 1823; H. MacDonald, 'Procuring Corpses: The English Anatomy Inspectorate 1842–1858', *Medical History*, 53 (2009): p. 388.

[78] LH/A17/1, 30 July 1811; Richardson, *Death, Dissection and the Destitute*, pp. 71, 104–5; MacDonald, 'Procuring Corpses', pp. 384–5.

[79] LH/A17/3, 19 November 1822.

whereupon the grave robbers threw dirt and stones at them, breaking the windows and injuring one of the patients. A few days later, body-snatchers broke into the dead house and stole the body of a young woman.[80] In December the patients discovered two grave robbers in the graveyard. Assisted by the house porter, the watchman and a constable, they attacked and captured them. The two men were sentenced to three months' hard labour.[81] Valentine informed the governors that the 'clamorous contentions' in the cemetery had opened the eyes of the patients to these proceedings and were most upsetting to them. He recommended better fencing around the burying ground as a means of preventing at least outsiders from stealing bodies.[82]

Valentine's complex ethical difficulties with grave robbers and fraudulent funerals aside, his most severe administrative problem was the standard one in all hospitals – nurses going out of the hospital, leaving their patients unattended for hours at a time. It was difficult to resolve, for the nurses had to shop for their food[83] and buy things for the patients such as tea and sugar which the medical officers ordered, but which the hospital did not supply. Valentine therefore allowed nurses to leave the hospital without written permission at 11 a.m.–12 noon and 3–4 p.m. He had considered providing them with vegetables so they would have fewer reasons for leaving their wards, which they did frequently, and often outside the permitted hours. At the same time, he felt that servants who were worked as hard as the nurses should be allowed to go out occasionally. They should not feel like prisoners, and also they needed to get some purer air – a reflection of the belief that emanations from the sick caused disease. He ordered that only one nurse from each ward could go out at a time, and he stopped the practice of the nurses fetching their own porter. Rather, he arranged to have it all brought in at a fixed hour by the steward, who pledged that he would see that none of the patients' porter would be given to the nurses to distribute, because when it was, they often drank it themselves.[84]

In 1824 a House Committee member, Mr Batson, lodged a major complaint against the nurses. They were, he said, 'from habit often so accustomed to the reverse of cleanliness that in spite of every regulation and constant admonition' they did no cleaning. Bandages and compresses were supposed to be washed in the wash house, but the nurses often washed them in the lobby sinks where the dishes and food were washed. The lobbies and water closets were filthy, and the new marble tubs were never properly cleaned. The gate porter often left his post in the charge of friends, who allowed spirits and food to be smuggled into the hospital while at the same time visitors carried hospital property out of the hospital. The

[80]    Ibid., 12 August 1823.

[81]    LH/A4/9, 3 December 1823.

[82]    LH/A17/3, 19 and 26 August, 2 September 1823.

[83]    Most hospitals gave their nurses some meat and bread, but none provided a full diet at this time.

[84]    LH/A17/3, 18 May 1824.

Nurses and assistant nurses continually went in and out of the hospital without the required written permission, and now claimed that it was their right to do so. Male patients loitered about in the women's wards.[85]

As well as indicating the lack of discipline, Batson's complaints illustrate the new concern with hygiene and the rising standard of living among the middle and upper classes, but his expectation that working-class women with their meagre incomes could achieve these standards was impracticable. Businesses supplied water to the city, and in poor areas often sold it by the jug. In one impoverished district of London, water was turned on for half an hour on three weekdays, and on Sundays for only five minutes.[86] Hospitals did not provide nurses with the time or resources needed for better hygiene. Most hospitals had baths in the basement for the patients and a movable tub on the floors. There was usually running water, but not hot running water. In 1828 at the Westminster, Dr Roe hesitated to prescribe warm baths for his patients because it took so much time for the nurses to carry the numerous pails of hot water through the halls and up the stairs to the wards.[87]

Linen was constantly stolen in all the hospitals. At the London, sheets disappeared from the laundry, the wards, and even from the beds, and since an assistant nurse had been prosecuted for stealing sheets, Valentine explained, even more had been taken: 17 disappeared all at once from one ward.[88] Literacy presented yet another problem. The assistant nurses were supposed to be able to read the prescriptions on the medicine bottles, but when Valentine advertised for literate women, not one in ten who applied was able to read and write. Nor was he convinced that it was necessary, or even possible, to obtain literate women who would be willing to do the 'laborious and disagreeable work' of assistant nurses. In any case, the Nurse, not the assistant nurse, administered medicines during the day. It was only between 11 p.m. and 6 a.m. that the night watchers gave out medications. During the night, things were so arranged that Valentine thought it highly unlikely that any serious mistake could happen. The governors insisted, however, that all nurses who were unable to read or write be dismissed.[89]

Under attack from Batson, Valentine became quite feisty. He declared he had made considerable improvements in the class of women whom he hired as nurses. It was easier to find respectable women among the illiterate than among those who knew how to write. Valentine expressed a standard view of nursing as a job of last resort when he explained how he had:

> obtained a class of servants very superior to the dirty, disgracefully dirty, unprincipled persons which, with a few exceptions, formed the great mass of

[85]    LH/A4/9, 2 June 1824.

[86]    E. Gauldie, *Cruel Habitations: A History of Working Class Housing 1780–1918* (London, 1974), pp. 73–7.

[87]    WH/A1/28, 13 August 1828.

[88]    LH/A17/3, 15 June 1824.

[89]    Ibid, 12 March 1822.

the hospital servants: but the supposed and perhaps real necessity of having assistant nurses who can write is attended with great disadvantage. Previously to this regulation honesty and cleanliness were the first requisites; now a number of each are refused, for a shabby, half-charactered woman who can write; I say half-charactered woman, for what really decent woman with a good character, and with something of an education, is driven to the necessity of submitting to the unseasonable, laborious, revolting, health destroying, character destroying, situation of a watcher at a hospital?[90]

## Moral Disorder: The Need for System, Regularity and Elevation of Character

The search for moral, or what we would call social, discipline at the London and Westminster was a constant theme in all the voluntary hospitals. Although hospitals were situated on the fringes of orderly society and were grouped together in official records with reformatories and prisons, moral disorder or 'lack of order and regularity', as the Westminster governors put it, was not limited to these peripheral institutions: it pervaded society as a whole. The search for better order was an overarching concern of the Victorian era. The upper classes, who were by no means restrained themselves, believed that a lack of moral restraint by individuals, and especially working-class individuals, was responsible for the riotousness and excesses of their time.[91] In London, rapid urbanization had produced large populations bred in the slums, brutalized by ignorance, squalor and drink. Almost 20 years of war on an unprecedented scale, the mass military mobilization, and after 1815, demobilization, helped to destabilize traditional social relationships built on lower-class deference. The fear of French revolutionary ideas, the massive changes caused by the burgeoning industrial revolution, and later, the campaigns to broaden male suffrage intensified the fear of the very real problem of disorder.[92]

It was an age of riots. High-ranking government officials considered it inevitable that their houses were occasionally sacked. The rioters were usually few, perhaps 50 men, but they could cause considerable mayhem and damage. For example, in March 1815, on the third reading of the Corn Laws, which levied tariffs on foreign grain in years of poor domestic harvests, making bread more expensive, a crowd of several thousand gathered outside the House of Commons to protest. A number moved off to attack the houses of those who supported the laws, including that of Lord Chancellor Eldon. They smashed windows, tore out railings and sacked the entrance hall and

---

[90] Ibid., 18 May 1824 (original emphasis).

[91] M.J. Wiener, *Reconstructing the Criminal: Culture, Law and Policy in England 1830–1914* (Cambridge, 1990), pp. 16–18, 26–7, 32–8, 45.

[92] M.J.D. Roberts, *Making English Morals: Voluntary Association and Moral Reform in England, 1787–1886* (Cambridge, 2004), ch. 2; M. Ackroyd et al., *Advancing with the Army: Medicine, the Professions and Social Mobility in the British Isles, 1790–1850* (Oxford, 2006), pp. 1–3.

an adjoining room, forcing Eldon to decamp through his garden into the grounds of the British Museum. With no police force in London until 1829, it was generally necessary to call in the militia or the army to stop riots. When the army appeared, Eldon managed to collar two of the men and told them that he would have them hanged, whereupon one responded that they were more likely to hang him. If the culprit was wrong in thinking Eldon would be hanged, he was right in thinking that he himself would go free. Typical of working-class loyalty, the soldiers who had restored order refused to testify against the rioters and the case was dismissed.[93]

The behaviour of many patients and hospital nurses demonstrated a similar riotous nature, lack of self-restraint and orderliness. For example, the administrators at St Thomas' reported in 1837 that 'turbulent conduct' was not infrequent among the patients. In the male venereal wards, disturbances or misbehaviour of some kind occurred at least once a week. When the hospital porters were unable to make the offenders leave, the steward called in the police. 'The steward visits the male, and the matron the female wards daily, to see that order is maintained,' the Charity Commissioners explained in 1837. 'No gaming, swearing, quarrelling, drinking, improper conversation or other immoral conduct' was allowed. Nevertheless, the house rules against smoking, gambling, swearing and fighting were frequently ignored. In several instances, the lives of sisters and nurses were threatened.[94]

In addition to riots within the hospitals, riots inflamed by fear of dissection and frequently blamed on the Irish sometimes began outside the hospital. In May 1832 a crowd of what hospital staff thought were 200 Irishmen invaded the Westminster and took away the body of a patient who had just died,[95] presumably to prevent it being dissected. Similarly, in 1847 Mrs Ward, Matron of King's College Hospital, claimed there had been times when 200–300 Irishmen had besieged the hospital.[96]

'The culture of the wards accepted anger and crudity as a part of every day occurrence,' Peter Stanley wrote of the surgeons,[97] but quarrels and outbursts of bad temper among the nurses were equally common. Some historians have suggested that hospital nurses in the earlier part of the nineteenth century have been unjustly maligned, and if they were callous, incompetent or dissolute, they were dismissed.[98] In fact, because it was so hard to recruit clinically experienced nurses, it was

---

[93]    D. Thomson, *England in the Nineteenth Century: 1815–1914* (London, 1950), pp. 12, 63–4; J. Stevenson, *Popular Disturbances in England 1700–1870* (London, 1979), pp. 190–91.

[94]    LMA/H09/GY/A71/1, pp. 677, 60.

[95]    LMA/H02/WH/A1/29, 8 May 1832.

[96]    KH/CM/M3, 26 March 1847.

[97]    Stanley, *For Fear of Pain*, p. 204.

[98]    See, for example, K. Williams, 'From Sarah Gamp to Florence Nightingale: A Critical Study of Hospital Nursing Systems from 1840 to 1897', in Davies (ed.), *Rewriting Nursing History*, pp. 57–8; A. Summers, 'Ministering Angels: Victorian Ladies and Nursing Reform', in G. Marsden (ed.), *Victorian Values: Personalities and Perspectives in Nineteenth Century Society* (2nd edn, London, 1998), p. 143.

standard practice to simply move quarrelsome, callous or incompetent nurses to a different ward. Dismissal was the last resort, and usually the result of sustained patient abuse or striking a patient. For example, in October 1857 the house surgeon at St George's asked Matron Frances Willey to suspend a night nurse because she treated the patients harshly and was unfit for her duties. Willey had already moved her twice to different wards for similar complaints.[99] There is no record of the night nurse's dismissal, leaving open the possibility that she was again moved to another ward. As well as demonstrating the difficulty of finding competent nurses, this policy shows how difficult it was for the matron, let alone the governors, to know what was going on at the level of individual patient care.

John Bell, the distinguished Scottish anatomist and surgeon, described the hospital atmosphere at the end of the eighteenth century as noisy and full of confusion and noxious air, creating 'agonies of mind' for the patients.[100] The historians Guenter Risse and John Harley Warner agreed:

> Keeping order in the wards, an ideal enshrined in countless hospital regulations, was usually difficult; thefts occurred, fights broke out, patients were punished for violating the rules, some inmates escaped, others had hysterical and epileptic fits or raved all night in their febrile delirium.[101]

The wards were not only noisy and chaotic, but also had an almost unbearable smell. As late as 1864 the Charity Commissioner who inspected St Thomas' reported that although the windows were always left open both day and night, the wards had 'an almost intolerable stench'.[102] Despite generous doses of cathartics and emetics, chamber pots were normally emptied only twice a day,[103] and the smells mingled with that of food cooking and rampant infection. It was not an atmosphere in which competent women of any class would choose to work.

## Conclusion

At the beginning of the nineteenth century, the general disorder in the voluntary hospitals was accepted, if not condoned, as a fact of life. It was no different from the disorder which permeated society as a whole, and with fewer acutely ill patients, fewer surgical procedures and fewer medical directives, unreliable nursing attendance did not make as much difference as it would later. However, the

---

[99]   SGH/MBG, 14 and 21 October 1857.

[100]   Stanley, *For Fear of Pain*, pp. 137–8.

[101]   G.B. Risse and J.H. Warner, 'Reconstructing Clinical Activities: Patient Records in Medical History', *Social History of Medicine*, 5 (1992): p. 191.

[102]   LMA/H01/ST/A44/2, pp. 65–6.

[103]   ST/A25; Florence Nightingale complained of this practice in 1878: BL 47760, fol. 30.

new medicine, and especially its supportive therapeutics, were heavily dependent on conscientious, intelligent nursing care. Patients with high fevers had to have their fluids replaced frequently, while a fresh tracheotomy patient could not be left in the care of a night watcher who might be sleeping, doing her washing or drinking the patients' stimulants. Equally important, a competent nurse had to know when to summon medical assistance. The old pre-industrial hospital culture simply could not support the new medicine. The disorderly and casual attitude which many old nurses took towards patient care undermined the effectiveness of the new medical practice. In the next chapter, we look more closely at the nature of hospital nursing services in the earlier nineteenth century and explore the structural problems which made it so difficult to make them more efficient.

# Chapter 2

# Hospital Nursing
# in the First Part of the Century

Nursing practice in the early nineteenth century was not meeting the requirements of the new medicine, and it was not easy to see how it could, or who should take responsibility for developing more efficient nursing. Doctors did not sit on the boards at the London and the three endowed hospitals, but they were governors at the other eight hospitals, and it was these doctors who first took the initiative. They did not try to reform nursing services in the sense of reorganizing them, but rather wrote stricter rules and tried unsuccessfully to get them enforced, gave gratuities for good behaviour, and raised salaries in the hope of attracting 'a superior type of woman'. For example, the Westminster raised its nurses' wages five times between 1809 and 1828, from £8 a year to 14 guineas.[1] Real wages increased during this period, so that the nurses were being much better recompensed.[2]

The founders and Sisters of St John's House, a nurses' training school founded in 1848 which we will cover in Chapter 7, were the first to recognize that the problems causing the inadequate nursing were structural; nursing needed to be rebuilt from the ground up. But it took until 1848 to appreciate this need. When Blizard and his colleagues reported to the House Committee at the London in 1818, they thought there was nothing wrong with the organization of the nursing department, but rather attributed the nursing problems to the matron's failure to enforce the rules. As well, they criticized her accounting and said she could not cope with the increased number of patients.[3] Scapegoating the matron became a standard response of both doctors and lay governors when stricter regulations and financial incentives failed to improve the nursing.

In this chapter we look at nursing practice in the early nineteenth century and explore three structural problems which made it almost impossible to deliver nursing care efficiently. The first problem was the matron's lack of authority and nursing knowledge. The second was the pre-industrial work ethic of the early

---

[1]  LMA/H02/WH/A1/25, 28 June 1809; 28 June 1815, 28 June 1816, 1 October 1817; LMA/H02/WH/A1/28, 23 April 1828.

[2]  See <http://www.bankofengland.co.uk/education/inflation/calculator/flash/index. htm> (accessed 10 July 2011); J. O'Donoghue, L. Goulding and G. Allen, 'Inflation since 1750', *Economic Trends*, 604 (March 2004): pp. 38–46, <http://www.statistics.gov.uk/ articles/economic_trends/ET604CPI1750.pdf> (accessed 10 July 2011). Overall, despite doubling between 1803–13, prices decreased from 1809 to 1828.

[3]  LH/A5/16, 19 December 1818.

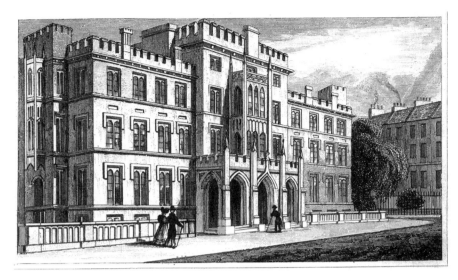

Figure 2.1     The New Westminster Hospital, 1834. This purpose-built hospital
               replaced the old, smaller hospital which was in what had formerly
               been a residential home. The new Hospital was in the Broad Sanctuary,
               across from Westminster Abbey and the Houses of Parliament. In
               some wards there was one bed partitioned off as a nurse's room.

*Source*: Wellcome Library, London, by kind permission.


nineteenth-century workforce. The third was the governors' utterly unrealistic
expectations of what, even with the best will in the world, nurses and matrons
could do. The records of all the teaching hospitals contain constant, and similar,
complaints revealing these basic weaknesses in the old nursing system.


**The Matron's Lack of Authority and the High Cost of Enforcing the
Regulations**

Like all women at the beginning of the nineteenth century, matrons lacked
legitimate public authority and needed the approval of the Weekly Board for any
major action such as hiring or firing, and in some hospitals, suspending her staff.
Critical as they were of their matron, even Blizard and his colleagues thought she
should have the power to suspend nurses.[4] As well, matrons became responsible
for increasingly sophisticated nursing services when they themselves had no
nursing experience. As a result, many nurses in the teaching hospitals failed to
comply with the rules and did not respect the matron's authority.

---

[4]     Ibid.

In 1835, shortly after moving into their new state-of-the-art hospital, the Westminster governors tried to address this problem by formulating minutely detailed nursing regulations which indicate, as is often the case with rules, where the problems lay. The rules, almost identical to those in the other teaching hospitals, also indicate the new medicine's growing dependence on skilled nursing. The nurses were to have a three-week probation period, be able to read handwriting, and be honest, sober and kind. They were responsible for the quietness and good order of the wards and for cleaning all the wards, rooms and passages of the hospital; they were to carry out the orders of the doctors and see that the patients took their medicine; they were to watch the patients, particularly during the night, so that they could report their symptoms to the medical officers at their next visit, or in the case of emergency, summon the apothecary or house surgeon; they were to assist those patients who were unable to wash themselves and see that the patients obeyed the hospital rules, especially with reference to bringing in or taking out food and liquor. Nurses themselves were never to take any provisions out of the hospital and were not to accept any money or gifts from the patients.[5]

The new regulations made little difference; the old problems persisted. In August 1836, the house surgeon found the night nurse in Northumberland Ward asleep several times, while Evans, the day nurse, had accepted a gift of meat from a patient. Night Nurse Macklin did not call the apothecary for an alarmingly ill patient until after he died. The two nurses were warned they would be discharged if they repeated these offences, but Macklin nevertheless only a month later accepted money from a patient's wife and also used abusive language to another patient.[6]

As well as these standard nursing problems, Matron Ann Cox's responsibilities were steadily increasing because all the hospitals were expanding, partly because London was growing so rapidly. In 1801 its population was 958,863, by 1841 it had doubled to 1,948,417, and by 1861 it contained 2,803,989 people.[7] Hospitals were also enlarging their bed capacity because the successes of the new medicine led more people to seek hospital care and doctors were admitting more acutely ill patients whom most hospitals had previously refused to accept.[8] When Cox started at the Westminster in 1818 there were less than 100 patients and only eight nurses and two female servants. Sixteen years later, in the new hospital there were 170 patients, 17 nurses and four female servants.[9]

Cox typically lacked the authority to effectively discipline those women who did not work out well; she could suspend offending nurses, but then had to wait for the Weekly Board to meet and decide whether to reprimand or dismiss the nurse.[10]

---

[5]   LMA/H02/WH/A34/1/1, pp. 9–10, 26–8, 31–2.

[6]   LMA/H02/WH/A1/31, 23 August, 25 October 1836.

[7]   See <http://www.londononline.co.uk/factfile/historical> (accessed 10 July 2011).

[8]   F.B. Smith, *The People's Health 1830–1910* (New York, 1979), pp. 278–81.

[9]   LMA/H02/WH/A1/30, 22 July 1834.

[10]   St Thomas' and Guy's were exceptions. There, the matron appointed and dismissed the nurses herself. LMA/H09/GY/A71/1, pp. 686, 737.

The Weekly Board was forced to reconsider this policy in March 1841 when the house visitors reported that the patients in St Matthew's and St Mark's Wards were extraordinarily insubordinate. Cox said the nurses kept the wards in a very dirty state, while the house surgeon said they were inattentive to their patients – a good illustration of the different responsibilities of the two officers: cleanliness of the wards for the matron, and nursing care for the surgeon. The day nurse allowed smoking, hard liquor and card playing, and permitted 'the grossest indecencies to be practiced on herself'. One patient was seriously assaulted because the others were so riotous and disorderly. The governors discharged the day and night nurses and gave the matron and secretary the power to conjointly summarily dismiss inferior servants in such cases.[11] The Westminster was unusual in giving the matron this partial power, a result of the need to act quickly rather than let such egregious disorder continue until the next Weekly Board meeting.

Some matrons, like Jane Morterras, did not attempt to enforce the rules, while others made only half-hearted attempts. St George's was unusual in finding a matron who conscientiously tried to implement the nursing regulations. In 1836 the hospital drew up more stringent nursing regulations and asked the new matron, Miss A. Steel,[12] to strictly enforce them. It was no coincidence that the increased attention to the nursing came just a year after the founding of the hospital's medical school. The 320 patients in the recently expanded hospital, and the closer superintendence the new rules required, greatly increased Steel's duties.[13]

When the new rules failed to improve the nursing, the board increased the responsibilities of the matron. They stressed that she was the mistress of the household and responsible for preserving its order and good government, and spelled out her duties in minute detail. She was to personally superintend the weighing and delivery of the 320 patients' meals, and ensure meals were served on time and that no food was wasted or embezzled. She was to give orders to the nurses on ward management; the rooms, bedding and linen were to be kept clean and well aired; she was to enforce hospital rules and see that medical orders were obeyed. She was to report offending nurses to the Weekly Board: in extreme cases, she could suspend nurses until the next Weekly Board, but only *if* the apothecary or house surgeon thought that the suspension would not inconvenience ward management. She was to superintend the sleeping apartments of the nurses, making sure that they got up and went to bed on time. Finally, she was to see that that the nurses and female servants did their work and treated the patients with tenderness and visitors with civility. In addition to all this, she had to keep all her inventories, submit written requests for all the articles required for the boardroom

---

[11]   LMA/H02/WH/A1/33, 16 and 30 March 1841. The inferior female servants were the assistant nurses and the kitchen staff; in the male wards, the porters and surgery man.

[12]   Sometimes spelled 'Steele'. The secretary's lack of interest in the correct spelling of the matron's name is another indication of her lack of importance in the hospital's administration.

[13]   SGH/MBG, 8 April 1836, 6 January, 23 November 1837.

and servants' tables, and was responsible for the laundry, linen and woollen stores. Female patients capable of working could help with needlework, rolling bandages or household duties.[14] The matron's regulations in the other teaching hospitals were essentially identical to those at St George's.

In a hospital of 320 beds, Steel's job was virtually impossible for one person.[15] Her conscientious but undiplomatic efforts to enforce the rules created resistance among her staff, causing the already high rate of turnover among them to increase. In July 1839, at a Weekly Board meeting two doctors moved that a committee be formed to inquire into the management of the nursing department and the causes of the high turnover.[16] The committee acknowledged that there had been a great lack of discipline in the hospital under the previous matron and that the new rules curtailed some of the former privileges of the nurses, in particular going out of the hospital without the matron's permission. They appreciated that Steel's strict enforcement of the rules led to considerable ill feeling towards her, but felt she had not enforced the regulations with the 'necessary discretion of temper', causing more than one competent nurse to leave. Worst of all, the night nurses and assistant nurses whom she presented to the board for hiring did not have enough nursing knowledge. The committee demanded a more efficient nursing service, asserting that the high rate of turnover among the nurses was inconvenient, and in many cases dangerous to the patients. The nursing department, they explained, was of 'vital importance to the well-doing of the patients'. The governors raised the wages of the night nurses, urged recruiting the head nurses from experienced nurses, and required the matron to make a written report each week on the state of her department, giving the names of every nurse or servant whom she suspended or who was about to leave.[17]

The nursing still did not improve,[18] but it was the suicide of Nurse Cheeseley, who killed herself by jumping off the hospital roof in December 1840, which led to Steel's downfall. Cheeseley was the head nurse of King's Ward and a long-standing hospital employee. Her conduct was characteristic of a senior nurse whom hospital governors in the first part of the century considered exemplary. Despite a problem with embezzling and a bad temper with her subordinates, the governors spoke of her 'constant kindness, integrity and good conduct'.[19] The unreformed manners of Cheeseley and Steel also illustrate what later Victorians would refer to as the undesirable 'tone' of hospital life in the earlier part of the century.[20]

---

[14]   Ibid., 5 July, 23 November 1837.

[15]   Ibid., 6 January 1837.

[16]   Ibid., 31 July 1839.

[17]   Ibid., 7 and 14 August 1839.

[18]   See, for example, SGH/MBG, 13 November, 25 December 1839, 15 and 22 July, 23 and 30 September, 14 October, 4 and 18 November, 30 December 1840.

[19]   SGH/MBG, 16 December 1840.

[20]   C. Helmstadter, 'A Real Tone: Professionalizing Nursing in Nineteenth-century London', *Nursing History Review*, 11 (2003): pp. 12–22, 24.

Some governors thought the matron's inept management had caused Cheeseley's suicide. They established a committee, chaired by the society doctor Sir Henry Holland, to investigate the matter. The committee found that Cheeseley's problems began when her assistant nurse accused her of the standard practice of embezzling hospital supplies – sending a basket of bread, meat, soap and candles out of the hospital. She admitted she had sent out some 'trifling articles', but said they actually belonged to her and were part of her wages. Shortly afterwards, an assistant nurse was fired for a similar offence and all the nurses were called into the board room and warned against taking hospital property. Three weeks later, Cheeseley's night nurse told her that the board was planning to charge her with stealing hospital supplies. This very much upset Cheeseley, although it turned out not to be true. Then she had a major fight with Steel. The matron reprimanded her for not allowing her assistant nurse to attend chapel in the morning on alternate Sundays as hospital regulations required. Both Steel and Cheeseley became very angry, with Cheeseley accusing the matron of spying on her. The committee described the quarrel as too much passion on the part of the matron and impertinence on the part of the Nurse. They thought this violent interchange had overpowered Cheeseley's reason, producing the excited state of mind which led to her suicide.

The coroner's inquest cleared Steel of the charge of causing Cheeseley's death. Steel had worried about moving Cheeseley to King's Ward because it was a larger ward on an upper floor. Because Cheeseley was elderly and infirm, Steel thought she might not be able to handle it. Steel had not asked the assistant nurse for information on Cheeseley's conduct, nor had she refused her permission to go out of the hospital, which was easily proved by the numerous tickets granting her leave of absence. While the committee agreed that the matron's severity was not responsible for the suicide, they believed she had not always treated Cheeseley with the kindness and consideration due to a nurse of such 'excellent character' and long employment in the hospital. On the contrary, Steel had reproved her frequently in an inconsiderate manner. The board felt it was essential that the senior nurses be treated with respect, otherwise they would not receive respect from their subordinates. 'The matron is a woman of clear understanding' who zealously enforces the rules of the hospital, the committee explained:

> but she does not appear always to have preserved that command of temper and language which is so necessary in the government of a large establishment. Unless such a temper is maintained by those in authority the service in the subordinate departments will never be performed well and cheerfully with that kindly feeling and mutual good will which might be expected to actuate all those who are engaged in a common work of pure Christian benevolence.[21]

---

[21]    SGH/MBG, 16 December 1840.

Like Batson's standards of cleanliness, the reformation of manners had penetrated the governors' class, but had not yet seeped into that of the matron and nurses.

Five days later, Steel offered to resign. She said it would be in the best interest of the hospital because she could not work in harmony with the physicians and surgeons, a clear indication that it was the doctors rather than the lay governors who were pushing for better nursing management. 'I have never spared myself; nor have my best exertions been wanting to uphold the laws and maintain the discipline committed to me,' Steel wrote. She explained that the odium of enforcing the new stricter rules had rested on her alone during her six years in office. She had hoped that she had a home in the hospital for the rest of her life, and did not know what lay before her in her 'solitary and unfriended condition'. She asked to stay until the middle of February, when she would formally tender her resignation.[22] In February, the reality of leaving both her job and her home led Steel to withdraw her offer to resign. She had been overexcited by Cheeseley's death and had felt unable to work with the medical officers, she wrote, but now that she had regained her composure and the hospital was running smoothly, she asked to remain as matron. She did not feel she was responsible for the high rate of turnover among the nurses, correctly pinpointing the harsh rules as a cause and urging the board to make the regulations less stringent. She pointed out again that she was solely dependent on her own exertions for her livelihood. Steel's pathetic appeal fell on deaf ears: the board insisted she resign.[23]

The new matron, Mrs Harriet Sophia Hains,[24] faced precisely the same difficulties as Steel – an indication that the problems were structural, rather than personal. The nurses exhibited all the standard problems: failure to do their work, going out of the hospital without permission, using intemperate language, quarrelling with the patients and the other nurses, stealing, getting drunk, taking money from patients and being unkind to them.[25] Hains forcefully emphasized her lack of authority to carry out her job. In June 1842 she told the board she was in an impossible situation with Head Nurse North, who 'behaved in a very insolent and violent manner' to her. The board had ignored the nurse's behaviour the previous month, and if she was not immediately discharged, Hains wrote, 'I cannot expect to receive that respect from those remaining under my management, nor to keep up that authority, so indispensable to the good order and government of my department.' The board discharged this nurse,[26] but Hains still could not establish her authority.

Her nurses knew that she could not dismiss them and that they could appeal over her head to the Weekly Board, which more often than not supported the

[22]    Ibid., 23 December 1840.
[23]    Ibid., 3 February 1841.
[24]    Hains is often called 'Harris' in the board minutes. We thank Dr Sue Hawkins for giving us her correct name.
[25]    For example, see SGH/MBG, 7 April, 8 and 15 September, 29 December 1841.
[26]    SGH/MBG, 15 June 1842.

nurse rather than the matron. Head Nurse Maria Dewar provides an example of a nurse who, because she was clinically experienced, was able to find three nursing jobs despite her refusal to accept her matron's direction. In September 1841 a young woman patient accused Dewar of inattention and using improper language. The St George's governors investigated, and decided the patient had trumped up these charges because Dewar had discovered friends were bringing her illicit provisions. In June 1842 another patient accused Dewar of treating him harshly. The governors thought this man was troublesome and irritable, and discharged him. The following December, however, Hains suspended Dewar for intoxication, disgraceful behaviour in her wards, and rudeness to the chaplain and house surgeon. Dewar persistently left the hospital when drunk despite Hains pointing out to her the impropriety of so doing. Dewar admitted the charges and was dismissed.[27] She then obtained a job as a head nurse at University College Hospital. In March 1845 the hospital was about to discharge Dewar and her night nurse for taking money from patients. Apparently, the committee thought better of it, for she remained a head nurse until October, when she was fired for insobriety.[28] Dewar then obtained a job as a night nurse at the Westminster, where, in October 1847, the secretary fired her for riotous conduct, drunkenness and assaulting one of the female patients.[29] Dewar took a major step down when she accepted a position as a night nurse, but nevertheless, despite a very poor work record, she was able to secure a third nursing job. Governors did indeed sometimes dismiss incompetent or dissolute nurses, but they did not blindly support their matrons when they reported a nurse for misbehaviour, and of course, the matron could not be aware of every misdemeanour.

Adding to the matron's heavy responsibilities, the new medicine was creating a growing need for her to understand nursing practice. In 1847 the doctors at the Middlesex Hospital, which had had a formal medical school since 1835, expressed their dissatisfaction with the nursing to their board. They were distressed by the understaffing, the high rate of turnover, and the wretched living and working conditions of their nurses. The nurses did not have regular meals, the night nurses were allowed only six hours out of the 24 for recreation and sleeping, and all were underpaid. Most importantly, many of the nurses were lacking in nursing knowledge, and their ignorance placed the patients, the doctors explained, 'in imminent danger'. The doctors were especially displeased with Matron Clementina Cookesley. Not only did they consider the nurses whom she hired incompetent and inefficient, but Cookesley herself admitted that she was not able to judge the nurses' qualifications nor was she competent to supervise their work.[30]

Pushed by the medical staff, in 1848 the governors made a major effort to improve the nursing. They added five nurses to their complement of 31, hired

27    Ibid., 18 September 1841, 15 June, 28 December 1842.
28    UCH/A2/1, 12 March, 8 October 1845.
29    LMA/H2/WH/A1/35, 19 October 1847.
30    MH/MBG, 23 February, 28 April, 24 August 1847.

scourers to relieve the nurses of some of their cleaning duties, and tried to upgrade the nurses' sleeping arrangements. Still, the nursing remained unsatisfactory, which the board attributed to the matron's mismanagement. Although they continually impressed on her the importance of hiring responsible nurses, they said, she persisted in hiring incompetent women.[31] The board was being unfair. Whether Cookesley understood nursing work or not, in London in the 1840s nurses who were both clinically experienced and respectable were few and far between.

Matters came to a head in 1849 when three board members complained forcefully about Cookesley and the board decided not to pay her the usual gratuity of £20 in addition to her £60 salary. Cookesley then wrote a letter to the board requesting a face-to-face hearing from which her three accusers would be excluded. She asked for a copy of the charges against her so that she could prepare her defence. She also asked that at least one friend accompany her to take notes and help her at the inquiry because, she said, 'As a woman, I am naturally unequal in such a matter to cope with men of ability and experience.' The board refused her request, saying it was 'highly improper and indecorous'. Unfair as this may seem to us now, in 1849 it was improper. The board was part of the male public sphere, and despite her position as a paid hospital officer, as a woman, the matron could not participate in the public arena. The governors recognized Cookesley's extensive duties and thought her salary inadequate for her heavy responsibilities, but nevertheless decided she did not deserve her £20 gratuity. After nine years of service, she was dismissed in May 1849.[32]

Few early nineteenth-century matrons could cope with both the extensive housekeeping and the doctors' increasing demands for more skilled nursing. Mrs Jane Nelson, matron of the London Hospital from 1833 to 1867, was an exception.[33] She was not a nurse, but she was an extremely able administrator and had strong support from her board, which Steel, Hains, and Cookesley did not. Together with House Governor Valentine, Nelson had at first been able to provide respectable and intelligent women as nurses, resulting in what her governors considered an excellent nursing service. However, as nursing became more sophisticated and labour-intensive, the shortage of competent nurses became more and more acute. By 1862 Nelson was 'in the greatest distress and anxiety' trying to provide extra nurses for acute cases. She had a certain number of respectable women upon whom she could call, but now, when she needed more nurses, such women were simply not to be found, and the problem was compounded by the fact that many women would not look after fever cases.[34] As nursing became more complex, more than respectability and intelligence was required; nurses needed experience, knowledge and good clinical judgement. By the 1860s the matron as well as the

---

[31]    Ibid., 18 and 25 January 1848, 3 February 1848.

[32]    Ibid., 30 January 1840, 6 February 1849, 22 and 30 May 1849.

[33]    S. Collins, 'Two Victorian Matrons of the London Hospital', *History of Nursing Society Journal*, 5/2 (1994/95): pp. 59–61.

[34]    LH/A4/12, 5 March 1862.

nurses needed to have nursing knowledge because, in the absence of ready-made skilled nurses, she had to be able to train inexperienced women.

In the endowed hospitals, the problems with the sisters appear to have been less severe, partly because these hospitals were able to pay more and provide better accommodation, and partly because the governors spent far more time looking after their extensive endowments than they did supervising internal hospital administration. Equally important, since doctors did not sit on their committees and therefore could not report the problems, the governors were usually unaware of specific nursing issues. In 1821 St Bartholomew's was an exception when the governors gave the sisters and nurses generous raises. The governors thought their low pay was the reason why they demanded tips from the patients and their visitors, a practice which the governors said led to 'undue partialities'. They hoped the better pay would stop this universal hospital custom.[35]

If the sisters in the endowed hospitals were somewhat superior, the assistant nurses were much the same because all hospitals drew on the same labour pool and paid them roughly the same wage.[36] In 1857, surgeon John Flint South, who had been associated with St Thomas' since 1813, complained of the high rate of turnover among the assistant nurses, whom he considered underpaid. Like Valentine, South appreciated that these women worked very hard, rarely sitting down five minutes together during the whole day.[37] In 1837 the Charity Commissioners ascribed the difficulty recruiting proper persons as assistant nurses, and especially night nurses, to the disagreeable and onerous nature of their work and its low pay. They also commented on their high rate of turnover when 'the necessary practical skill and experience are attained fully only after long service',[38] but as we will see, few assistant nurses had long service.

The 'order and regularity' which the sisters maintained in their wards was also similar to that in the unendowed hospitals. The rigid fixed schedules which by the end of the century were the stamp of the new nursing did not exist. Rather, the old pre-industrial sense of time prevailed. In 1837 at St Bartholomew's, breakfast and dinner, which were prepared in the main kitchen, were served at 8–9 a.m. and 1–2 p.m. respectively, but the two meals the nurses prepared in the ward kitchens were served at their convenience. At Guy's, the patients got up when they pleased. At St Thomas', they could get up when they wished as long as they were dressed for chapel at 9.15 a.m.[39] As late as the 1870s, the sisters at Guy's had no fixed hour of

---

[35]    SBH/Ha1/17, 3 July 1821.

[36]    The cash payments differed considerably, but were usually compensated for by various payments in kind. See B. Abel-Smith, *A History of the Nursing Profession* (London, 1960), pp. 279–80.

[37]    South, *Facts Relating to Hospital Nurses*, pp. 11–12, 16–17.

[38]    LMA/H09/GY/A71/1, p. 674.

[39]    Ibid., pp. 677, 738.

work; as long as they were in the wards for the doctors' rounds, they could come and go at will.[40]

What was the nursing knowledge which the doctors at St George's and the Middlesex felt so many nurses grievously lacked? In the eighteenth century it was assumed that there was none: anyone could nurse the patients. Well into the second half of the nineteenth century, convalescent patients were ordered to assist the nurses with both cleaning and what we would now call nursing duties. In 1858, Florence Nightingale, whose standards were higher than those of most nurses of her time, deprecated the common practice of delegating unpleasant parts of nursing care such as enemas to patients. But even she thought the convalescents should help with the lighter cleaning, lifting patients, and giving and emptying bedpans.[41]

An investigation at St George's as late as 1867 illustrates the way patients did a good deal of the nursing. Elizabeth Evans, a patient in Wellington Ward, gave birth to a baby who died shortly after being sent home. Mrs Baily and Mrs Tracy, the day and night nurses, told the committee that two patients, Miss Hill and Jane Besley, had helped them care for the baby. At first, Hill took entire charge of the infant, but after a day or two it proved more than she could manage, so Besley took over. The nurses, who, she said, could not have been kinder to both mother and child, 'were only too glad of getting it to themselves and even showed an unwillingness to part with it'. They bottle-fed the baby with warm milk and gruel. After about a week, it developed thrush.[42] The doctors ordered borax and honey, which Hill applied to the baby's mouth. The baby was sent home in a clean state, wearing hospital clothes but suffering from thrush and the diarrhoea from which it died.[43]

Apart from applying solutions such as borax and honey, what other care did nurses give (or delegate to patients) in the first part of the century? Bleeding, leeching, vomiting, purging, enemas, salivating and blistering formed the basis of the old therapeutics. By mid-century, low diets and bleeding in particular had become the mark of an old-fashioned practitioner; cathartics and diuretics remained essentials in the medical armamentarium, but doctors used the drugs in smaller doses. Nevertheless, what historian Charles Rosenberg called 'the inertia of traditional practice' meant that the old therapeutics persisted.[44] Nurses administered all of these treatments except bleeding with the lancet. In the early nineteenth century they would often have to apply 50–60 leeches to one patient

---

[40]    *PP*, 1890–91, vol. 13, p. 3.

[41]    Florence Nightingale, 'Introducing Female Nurses into Military Hospitals', in L.R. Seymer (ed.), *Selected Writings of Florence Nightingale* (New York, 1954), pp. 56–8.

[42]    A fungal infection, characteristically of the mouth.

[43]    SGH/Minutes of Nursing Committee, Miscellaneous Committee Book, 16 and 23 November 1867.

[44]    C.E. Rosenberg, 'The Therapeutic Revolution', in M.J. Vogel and C.E. Rosenberg (eds), *The Therapeutic Revolution: Essays in the Social History of Medicine* (Philadelphia, PA, 1979), pp. 7–9, 15, 18. See also Stanley, *For Fear of Pain*, p. 173.

and see that all the leeches bit. The bleeding continued for several hours after the leeches dropped off, and the blood was often kept flowing longer by applying warm fomentations or a poultice.[45] Leeches were sometimes applied in relays, 15–20 at a time, so that the blood was kept constantly oozing for 24–36 hours.[46] It was often difficult to stop the bleeding, so nurses had to watch for this eventuality.[47] In the early nineteenth century, emetics[48] were second only to bloodletting in frequency of use because vomiting was believed to control vascular action, diminish inflammation and restore natural secretions.[49] Nurses gave the emetics and tended the vomiting patient.

Florence Nightingale described the disease process in 1859 as 'more or less a reparative process … an effort of nature to remedy a process of poisoning or decay, which has taken place weeks, months, sometimes years beforehand unnoticed'.[50] Because disease was an effort at repairing the body, it was important to support the symptoms which were thought to be part of the healing process. Vomiting, diarrhoea and all kinds of skin rashes and open sores were seen as wholesome efforts of the body to rid itself of the morbid poisons derived from miasmas or from a poor or immoral lifestyle. Even Dr George Johnson, a physician to King's College Hospital and one of the new academic and scientific practitioners, believed strongly in supporting the eliminative process in cholera despite its violent diarrhoea. In the 1850s he was giving cholera patients half an ounce of castor oil every half hour.[51]

Doctors 'blistered' their patients or deliberately created open sores because they were believed to attract the morbid excitement from one part of the body to themselves, allowing it to escape through the open wound. A blister at the nape of the neck, for example, was believed to reduce cerebral inflammation.[52] Blisters usually consisted of poultices made with mustard or the more potent Spanish

---

[45]   Poultices consisted of a soft mass made usually of bread, linseed or mustard, usually warmed, and wrapped in linen or muslin. They were applied to the skin or a wound to relieve pain, to keep leech bites bleeding or as a counter-irritant.

[46]   R.J. Graves, *Clinical Lectures 1834–35 and 1836–37* (Philadelphia, PA, 1838), pp. 62–3.

[47]   C.J. Pfeiffer, *The Art and Practice of Western Medicine in the First Half of the Nineteenth Century* (London, 1985), pp. 47–9; R.J. Graves, *Clinical Lectures on the Practice of Medicine*, ed. Dr Nelligan [1848] (2 vols, London, 1864), vol. 1, p. 148; G.B. Risse, *Hospital Life in Enlightenment Scotland: Care and Teaching at the Royal Infirmary of Edinburgh* (Cambridge, 1986), pp. 202–17.

[48]   Emetics are drugs used to induce vomiting.

[49]   Pfeiffer, *The Art and Practice of Western Medicine*, pp. 198–201.

[50]   Florence Nightingale, *Notes on Nursing: What It Is, and What It Is Not* [1859] (London, 1980), pp. 5–6. See also Risse, *Hospital Life in Enlightenment Scotland*, p. 239.

[51]   Book review of George Johnson, *On Epidemic Diarrhoea and Cholera*, in *British and Foreign Medical-Chirurgical Review*, 16 (1855): p. 114.

[52]   Stanley, *For Fear of Pain*, pp. 53–7; Rosenberg, 'Therapeutic Revolution', p. 23.

fly (cantharides). Nitrous acid or another caustic was occasionally used instead of the bandage-type poultice-blister. Blisters were also standard treatments for fevers, and could be used as stimulants to promote the energies of the nervous and circulatory systems or of particular organs. In 1801, Dr Richard Weekes thought he was in the minority when he condemned 'the common practice ... to blister from head to foot'.[53] In the earlier part of the century, blisters were left on for 12, 18 or 24 hours, and when they were removed, the whole epidermis[54] of the blistered part was torn away, leaving a raw, irritable surface from which large quantities of serum and pus drained for several days, to the great torture of the patient. The extensive ulcerations could be very difficult to heal, and Robert James Graves, the great Irish clinician, described these blisters as the patients' greatest trial and an almost insupportable agony.[55] Graves therefore recommended 'flying blisters' as stimulants – blisters to the chest, stomach area, inside of the legs and thighs which were applied for only two to three hours[56] – another enormous increase in the nurses' work. Poulticing was a major method of dressing blisters and surgical and other wounds, and was the work of the assistant nurses, not the sisters. As late as the 1870s it was still standard for a nurse to make 14–15 poultices a day because nearly all the wounds became infected and required dressing.[57]

Enemas were especially important in the days before intravenous therapy, as this was the only way food and fluids could be given when patients could take nothing by mouth, as in the case of Henry Franklin. Usually nurses gave one to two ounces at a time every one to two hours. There were many mixtures. Beef tea mixed with milk was one standard recipe, and a half ounce of beef tea, half an ounce of brandy, an egg yolk and a teaspoon of arrowroot another. Then there were medicinal enemas, for example starch or arrowroot with a few drops of opium to prevent diarrhoea.[58]

---

[53]   Ford (ed.), *A Medical Student at St Thomas' Hospital 1801–1802* (London, 1987), p. 66.

[54]   The top layer of the skin.

[55]   Graves, *Clinical Lectures on the Practice of Medicine* [1848], vol. 1, pp. 158–61; J. Cheyne, 'Medical Report of the Hardwicke Fever Hospital for the Year Ending on the 31st March 1817', *The Dublin Hospital Reports and Communications in Medicine and Surgery*, vol. 1 (1818): pp. 25–6.

[56]   Graves, *Clinical Lectures on the Practice of Medicine* [1848], vol. 1: pp. 149–50, 155–6. For a detailed description of nursing methods of applying blisters, see M. Libster and Sister B. McNeil, *Enlightened Charity: The Wholistic Nursing Care, Education and Advices Concerning the Sick of Sister Matilda Coskery 1799–1870* (West Lafayette, IN, 2009), pp. 194–8.

[57]   Z. P. Veitch, *Handbook for Nurses for the Sick* (London, 1870), pp. 25–7, 30; Sister Casualty, 'A Reformation', *St Bartholomew's League News* (May 1902): pp. 134–8; South, *Facts Relating to Hospital Nurses*, p. 16.

[58]   See, for example, KH/M5/MS, 17 February 1853; Veitch, *Handbook for Nurses for the Sick*, pp. 23–6.

Mercury compounds were a mainstay of drug treatment. As one doctor stated in 1824, 'There are but few diseases in which it [mercury] is not most liberally administered.'[59] Salivating treatment – giving mercury to the point where the patient suffered mercury poisoning, spitting two and a half to three pints of saliva a day – was considered a cure for syphilis.[60] Sisters in the salivating or foul wards were given hardship pay. For example, at St Bartholomew's in 1802 they received £52 16s.7d. a year, compared to sisters of clean wards at £32 6s. 10d. and sisters of the operation wards at £37 16s. 10d.[61]

Effective nurses had to have clinical experience with these procedures, giving them the necessary professional judgement. 'There are many nurses who are extremely attentive, but inexpert and injudicious, and their ill judged attentions are frequently prejudicial to the patient,' Graves told his students in the mid-1830s. Before antibiotics and intravenous therapy, fevers were higher and lasted much longer – two to three weeks or more. Experience dealing with delirious patients and 'the mere handling of a patient', Graves continued:

> the moving of him from one bed to another, the simple act of giving him medicine or drink, the changing of his sheets and linen, the dressing of his blisters, and a thousand other offices, can be performed with advantage only by an experienced nurse …. In the advanced stages of fever the services of a properly qualified nurse are inestimable.[62]

In 1818, a typical regimen of nursing care for a febrile patient with a concussion of the brain consisted of leeches and cold applications to the head, fomentations to the legs, a blister at the nape of the neck, and mild mercurials and ipecac.[63] The old therapeutics obviously demanded an enormous amount of time-consuming nursing care and considerable clinical knowledge and judgement. When frequent feeding and fluids, the making of all disposable dressings, pain control, new standards of cleanliness, a major increase in the number of operations, post-anaesthetic care and conscientious patient assessment were added to the nurses' duties, one can see why the assistant nurses rarely had a chance to sit down, as South pointed out.

---

[59]    Pfeiffer, *The Art and Practice of Western Medicine*, pp. 201–6.

[60]    Clark-Kennedy, *The London*, vol. 1, pp. 40–41.

[61]    N. Moore, *The History of St. Bartholomew's Hospital* (2 vols, London, 1918), vol. 2, pp. 769–72.

[62]    Graves, *Clinical Lectures on the Practice of Medicine* [1848], vol. 1, pp. 114–19, citation on p. 115. Fever patients were often moved to a different bed once a day in order to escape the dangerous noxious emanations which they were believed to emit and which permeated the bed. It was thought that healthy persons produced these harmful secretions, but those who were sweating from fever produced far more.

[63]    Cheyne, 'Medical Report of the Hardwicke Fever Hospital', p. 27. Ipecac is an emetic.

## The Pre-industrial Work Ethic and the Reformation of Manners

The pre-industrial work ethic of the nurses and other hospital servants, although disappointing to hospital governors, was characteristic of the early nineteenth-century workforce as a whole. Historian Richard Price demonstrated that securing 'a general obedience and consent to the rhythm of capitalist production' was the major task of early industrialists. He identified the two central challenges as regular attendance at work and getting the work itself actually done,[64] precisely hospital nurses' two main problems: failure to show up for work or leaving their wards unattended, and when they were in the wards, failure to do their work, what the governors termed 'inattention to their duties'.

The industrialists fought an uphill battle to improve attendance at work. In the old agrarian society, working time depended on the season of the year, the light, the weather and so on, but in the new industrial society, time became controllable, a commodity, a fundamental organizational principle of working life. Strict timetables which made efficient use of all the worker's time were also considered one way of elevating character. Only religious orders had controlled activities through the day with such exactitude as did the Victorians.[65] The early nineteenth-century workforce, used to determining its own hours, did not adjust easily to the strict factory schedules, harsh discipline and the declining number of holidays which the Industrial Revolution introduced. Many workers observed St Monday; cotton spinners in the first half of the century frequently did not appear for work on Tuesdays as well. Traditionally, many workers worked just long enough to maintain their usual standard of living. In one shoe factory in Northampton, the workers, like the sisters at Guy's, came and went at will; they only began appearing regularly when their employers locked them out when they arrived late.[66]

The nurses' high rate of turnover was characteristic. The supply of skilled labour was extremely problematic; in trades like engineering, the turnover rate could be as high as 100 per cent a year. The nurses' disorderly behaviour was also typical of the early nineteenth-century workforce as a whole. William Brown, a flax mill owner in Dundee at the turn of the century, explained that his factory often fell into disorder. Because maintaining social discipline among his workers was his central problem, he inspected every aspect of his factory every day, but only occasionally looked at the number of workmen employed,

---

[64]    R. Price, *Labour in British Society: An Interpretative History* (London, 1986), pp. 37–8.

[65]    L. Davidoff, *The Best Circles: Women and Society in Victorian England* (Totowa, NJ, 1973), pp. 34–5; G. Davison, *The Unforgiving Minute: How Australia Learned to Tell Time* (Melbourne, 1993), pp. 2–5, 13–16, 22–3; E.P. Thompson, 'Time, Work-discipline and Industrial Capitalism', *Past and Present*, 38 (1967): pp. 60–63, 70–76.

[66]    J. Voth, *Time and Work in England 1750–1830* (Oxford, 2000), pp. 268–270; H. Perkin, *Origins of Modern English Society* (London, 1969), pp. 128–31; Price, *Labour in British Society*, p. 110.

their character, attendance or even their wages. In the same way, hospitals did not preserve systematic records of nurses and sisters until the 1890s.[67] Indeed, as Price wrote: 'The problem of industrial discipline was inseparable from the wider problem of social discipline generally.'[68] Irregular attendance and disorder created inefficiencies and lower profits for factory owners. In the hospitals, with their increasingly acutely ill patients, it was a much more serious problem, for patients' lives often depended on regular attendance by a skilled nurse.

Moral restraint, moral reform, character elevation, civility or the reformation of manners – whichever nineteenth-century term one prefers to use but which we in the twenty-first century call 'work discipline' and 'social order' – was essential if nursing was to become efficient. Historians Arthur Burns and Joanna Inness demonstrated that in this period, all reform carried a moral connotation, whether it was what we now in the twenty-first century consider moral – such as being a conscientious, honest worker – or institutional – such as parliamentary reform. In the nineteenth century, reform could mean redesigning laws and institutions or correcting personal moral failings; the two were interactive. Moral and institutional reforms were integrally intertwined: institutions were corrupt because of the moral failings of their personnel, and corrupt institutions corrupted the individuals within them.[69]

Anne Marie Rafferty, in her book on nursing knowledge since the mid-nineteenth century, wrote that: 'Nursing education has been characterized by the inculcation of moral values and virtues rather than intellectual prowess.'[70] This emphasis on moral and personal values began in the late eighteenth century. In the second half of the nineteenth century, the emphasis on improving moral character lessened in most occupations, and nursing was unusual in maintaining this emphasis for so long. In the first half of the nineteenth century, however, moral development was the normal understanding of education: education meant moral and intellectual discipline, imparting values and building character. For all members of the working classes, not simply nurses, character rather than learning was the key to successful employment. Valentine was expressing a mainstream preference when he preferred good character to literacy in the nurses he hired. Nor was the emphasis on development of moral character restricted to working-class persons. For example, in the first part of the nineteenth century 'medical education' meant developing the medical student's morals, while 'medical improvement' was the term used for what we now call 'medical education'.[71]

---

[67]    B. Craig, 'A Guide to Historical Records in London, England and Ontario, Canada c. 1800–c.1950', *Canadian Bulletin of Medical History*, 8 (1991): pp. 274–5, 277.

[68]    Price, *Labour in British Society*, pp. 37–9.

[69]    A. Burns and J. Innes, 'Introduction', in A. Burns and J. Innes (eds), *Rethinking the Age of Reform: Britain 1780–1850* (Cambridge, 2003), pp. 1–3, 39–40, 66.

[70]    Rafferty, *Politics of Nursing Knowledge*, p. 1.

[71]    'Medical Education', p. 147; D. Vincent, *Literacy and Popular Culture: England 1750–1914* (Cambridge, 1989), pp. 64–5.

Moral and religious instruction was at the heart of the education which the voluntary religious societies, with increasing help from the state, were extending to the poor in the 1830s and 1840s. Teachers emphasized preservation of social order, protecting property and preventing riots and disturbances – precisely the major concern of hospital administrators. In the town and country slums where the new teachers worked, this was absolutely necessary because the children had no sense of discipline or respect for their teachers. As in the hospitals, violence was not uncommon; pupils and their parents frequently assaulted teachers.[72] Working-class children usually attended school irregularly for only two or three years, and as with the nurses, punctuality was infrequent, with the teachers as unpunctual as the children.[73]

In the case of the nurses, punctuality was essential for good practice as well as a sign of good moral character. The new medicine depended heavily for its success on timely patient assessment, regular feeding, prompt removal of blisters, checking that leech bites did not bleed too long and so forth. It was simply not possible to do this without adherence to a schedule. However, just as it was unrealistic to expect hospital nurses to maintain the same standards of cleanliness as did upper-class women with their numerous servants, it was extremely difficult for early nineteenth-century nurses to be punctual when they had no watches, there were few clocks in the hospitals and they depended on a series of bells to tell them when it was time to get the beer, bread, or breakfasts and dinners.[74]

There were also political aspects to moral reform, which historian Martin Wiener summarized when he wrote: 'the need to build the working class character permeated virtually every field of understanding of human nature, society and public policy-making'. He argued that much of early Victorian social policy stemmed from fear of uprisings and can be interpreted as a series of efforts to contain and master what the upper classes considered the unregulated passions and instincts of the lower classes.[75] Another historian, Michael Roberts, demonstrated that this drive for moral reform was a major force in English society from the 1780s until the 1880s. He indicated it was part of an effort to correct a social order which the new market economy had destabilized.[76] Hospital governors' concern with preventing riotous behaviour and building character in the nurses reflected

---

[72]   A. Tropp, *The School Teachers: The Growth of the Teaching Profession in England from 1800 to the Present Day* (Westport, CT, 1977), p. 10.

[73]   J.H. Rigg, *National Education in its Social Conditions and Aspects, and Public Elementary School Education English and Foreign* (London, 1873) pp. 292–305, 317–18; G. Sutherland, *Elementary Education in the Nineteenth Century* (London, 1971), pp. 18–19; F.M.L. Thompson, *The Rise of Respectable Society* (London, 1988), pp. 144–50; J. Rule, *The Labouring Classes in Early Industrial England, 1750–1850* (London, 1986), p. 15.

[74]   LMA/H01/ST/A25.

[75]   Wiener, *Reconstructing the Criminal*, pp. 44–5.

[76]   Roberts, *Making English Morals*, pp. 13–18, 26–7, 32–8, 45.

the wider concern with moral reform, but was intensified by the demands of the new medical practice.

Some historians have interpreted the mid-nineteenth-century nursing reforms as having less to do with improving nursing care than with imposing middle-class values on the working classes.[77] It has even been suggested that doctors' complaints against nurses 'can also be understood as a smokescreen for their own clinical failure'.[78] In contrast, our research has revealed that in the early nineteenth century, doctors, hospital governors and matrons were primarily interested in better patient care, and that their complaints, as well as those of numerous hospital patients, were well founded. We must keep this in mind when we consider revisionist attempts to defend the old nurses against Dickens's fictional Sarah Gamp stereotype. Hospitals were very different organizations from the factories which the Industrial Revolution spawned or the elementary schools which the state was subsidizing, but hospital nurses came from the same society and shared the same culture. It would be very surprising if they had not shared the same work ethic.

## The Governors' Unrealistic Expectations of the Nurses and Matron

The demands hospital governors placed on their matrons were hardly realistic, as the experiences of Steel and Cookesley illustrated. It was also unreasonable to place a woman with no clinical experience in charge of a ward in a teaching hospital, but it was the assistant and night nurses who were placed in the most impossible situation. For example, in November 1827 the Westminster's Weekly Board reprimanded a nurse who had not reported a patient who was taken ill at 8 p.m. until 11 p.m. She explained that she had not seen any symptoms until 10 p.m.; when she went to report to the apothecary, he was out attending a private patient and did not return until 11 p.m. The apothecary said the nurse had not been negligent, but was simply inexperienced. Nevertheless, the governors told the nurse that if she was not experienced enough to note the symptoms of every patient, she could not be retained. Upon any future neglect, they said, ignoring the apothecary's statement, she would be immediately dismissed.[79] Held accountable by the governors for everything that happened in the ward as well as the cleanliness of patients and the hospital plant as a whole, responsible for assessing the patients' symptoms and administering their treatments, looked down

---

[77]   See, for example, K. Williams, 'From Sarah Gamp to Florence Nightingale', pp. 55–8; Rafferty, *Politics of Nursing Knowledge*, pp. 1–5, 9–13; A. Summers, *Angels and Citizens: British Women as Military Nurses 1854–1914* (London, 1988), pp. 38–40; A. Summers, 'The Mysterious Demise of Sarah Gamp: The Domiciliary Nurse and her Detractors c. 1830–1860', *Victorian Studies*, 33 (1989): pp. 376–8, 385–6.

[78]   Rafferty, *Politics of Nursing Knowledge*, p. 11.

[79]   LMA/H02/WH/A1/29, 4 November 1827.

upon as menials, working under dreadful conditions with a high rate of turnover, little general education and no training in nursing, these women were expected to perform nursing duties which required discipline, experience and knowledge.

## Conclusion

Given these structural problems, how well did the old nurses implement the new therapeutics? Like the managers of the new factories, who were of necessity less interested in the details of production than in maintaining order in the workplace, both lay and medical governors were forced to pay less attention to the level of patient care which nurses delivered than to the respectability and good order in their wards. It was not possible to deliver good care in a riotous ward, and in any case, good nursing care was frequently less visible than the cleanliness, neatness and quiet of the wards which was historically the nurses' primary responsibility.

We have no first-hand reports from the nurses themselves. With the exception of the kitchen maids, the assistant and night nurses had the lowest status of any hospital employee. Their superiors did not consider them worthy of special notice, while the nurses themselves were often illiterate, and at best insufficiently educated to produce their own records. The only instance where we found comments on the performance of a nursing staff as a whole was in 1824, when the House Committee at the London Hospital awarded gratuities and raises to their nurses. There are two important caveats to this example. First, nursing at the London was probably better than in the other hospitals because there was a resident professional administrator who took a lively interest in the nurses. Secondly, because doctors did not sit on the board at the London, the men who made the decisions had no direct experience of ward practice.

The House Committee gave bonuses to seven of eight head nurses. Isabella Anderson was described as the 'most industrious and the best nurse in the house'. Ann Maddy, who had one of the heaviest wards, was 'very attentive, highly respectable in character and conduct' and very humane. Sarah Lowe was 'a very good servant' who kept her ward particularly neat and her patients in good order. Catherine Wills was 'exceedingly kind and attentive to her patients', with 'a good character and an obliging disposition'. Francis McLean was 'very kind to her patients, obliging in her behaviour', and kept her wards neat and clean. Anne Filmer had an excellent character and was 'very well disposed and kind to her patients'. Susan Jewell was the only nurse commended for a clinical skill: she was very attentive to her patients, particularly with reference to administering medicines.[80] From a lay perspective, the ideal nurse in the earlier part of the century emerges as respectable, attentive and kind to patients, and able to keep good order in her wards.

[80]   LH/A4/9, 3 March 1824.

Compared to seven of the eight Nurses, only three of the more numerous assistant nurses were commended, and all that was said about them was that Mary Davis and Mary Black were two of the best assistant nurses in the hospital, while Ann Brofey was a steady, quiet, hard worker.[81] This is not to assert that no assistant nurses in the early part of the century had nursing knowledge. The surgeon Sir James Paget described the assistant nurses at St Bartholomew's in the 1830s as 'for the most part rough, dull, unobservant and untaught women', but he thought they were 'kindly and careful' and carried out medical orders.[82] He also remembered a sister in the same period as 'rough-tongued, scolding, frequently rather tipsy, yet very watchful and very helpful'.[83] Florence Nightingale thought, with some justification, that doctors were the worst judges of nurses because they were in the wards so seldom, and the nurses usually put on their best front when they were.[84] Nevertheless, doctors' views cannot be entirely dismissed. That the doctors at St George's complained of the inadequate nursing knowledge of many of their assistant and night nurses indicates that they had some skilled nurses whom they valued.

Relying on the received wisdom, Peter Stanley asserted that there is abundant evidence of competent nursing before 1860. He specifically mentions St Thomas' matron's claim that she had improved the type of sisters employed since 1816. He lists two nameless nurses at Charing Cross Hospital who gave unremitting care to a patient for three days, a St George's nurse who understood the care of aneurysms, and mentions two other sisters by name, Mrs Clarke and Mary Owen.[85] Mrs Clarke was the widow of a colleague of Sir Astley Cooper, a pre-eminent surgeon. Cooper found her a position as a sister at Guy's, where she remained for almost the rest of her life, but became addicted to drink, despite the fact, Cooper said, that she had previously been 'a most excellent woman, and really a genteel person'.[86] Mary Owen, Sister Rahere at St Bartholomew's, is frequently cited. Sir James Paget remembered her in the 1830s showing an ignorant house surgeon the location of the post-tibial artery. She worked at St Bartholomew's for 39 years, first as a nurse and then a sister. On her death in 1848, she left the hospital £250.[87] Apart from the 1824 London Hospital record cited above, we have found only a

---

[81]   Ibid.

[82]   C.T. Dent, 'History of Nursing at St. George's Hospital', *St George's Hospital Gazette*, 2/14 (1894): pp. 83–4.

[83]   G. Yeo, *Nursing at Bart's: A History of Nursing Service and Nurse Education at St. Bartholomew's Hospital, London* (London, 1995), p. 20.

[84]   BL 45805, fols 159–61.

[85]   Stanley, *For Fear of Pain*, pp. 145–6.

[86]   B.B. Cooper, *The Life of Sir Astley Cooper, bart.* (2 vols, London, 1843), vol. 1, p. 148.

[87]   W. Hector, 'Nursing', in V.C. Medvei and J.L. Thornton (eds), *The Royal Hospital of St. Bartholomew* (London, 1974), p. 251; Yeo, *Nursing at Bart's*, p. 20; SBH/Ha1/20, 13 June 1848.

few other references to individual clinically skilled head nurses/sisters, and none to assistant or night nurses. At St Thomas' in 1819, Golding praised Mrs Wilcox, the sister of the lithotomy ward who, after almost 40 years' service, was invaluable because of her 'great experience, acknowledged skill and tried humanity'.[88] John Flint South mentioned four outstanding sisters, one of whom was Mrs Wilcox.[89] A few outstanding examples do not make a skilled nursing workforce; these sisters were so memorable because they were exceptions.

Because many nurses were not up to the demands of caring for acutely ill patients in the new world of clinical medicine, teaching hospitals commonly relied on medical students for nursing care of the dangerously ill. Guy's Hospital had two 'clinical wards', one male and one female, for patients who required 'constant and extreme watchfulness'. The clinical lecturer attended daily with his 20–30 pupils, and each day two pupils were selected to care for these patients from 10 a.m. until the evening.[90] There were similar clinical wards at St Thomas'.[91] On occasion, the medical students stayed all night with the patient,[92] but medical students had many other responsibilities and could not be used as full-time nurses. Other solutions had to be found – ones which directly tackled the huge deficiencies in hospital nursing.

[88]   Golding, *An Historical Account*, pp. 228–9.

[89]   South, *Facts Relating to Hospital Nurses*, p. 14.

[90]   LMA/H9/GY/A71/1, pp. 739–40.

[91]   LMA/H01/ST/C2/1 and 2.

[92]   R.B. Todd, *Clinical Lectures on Certain Acute Diseases* (Philadelphia, PA, 1860), p. 133.

Chapter 3

# The Ward System: A Doctor-driven Reform

In 1880, John Braxton-Hicks, the noted Guy's Hospital obstetrician, described the three nursing systems then in existence: the ward system, the oldest and most prevalent, and the one he thought the best; the training institution, and the Anglican Sisters' centralized system.[1] He was writing in response to the famous and most researched nineteenth-century nursing dispute, the 'Crisis at Guy's', touched off when Matron Margaret Burt introduced the centralized system. The medical staff vigorously resisted Burt's innovations and tried unsuccessfully to have her dismissed.[2] In this chapter we examine the ward system which the Guy's doctors so ardently defended later in the century. It was the earliest reorganization of hospital nursing, developing over the first half of the nineteenth century in response to the more active role which doctors were playing in the teaching hospitals. It was also known as the 'sister system' because it made the ward sister its lynch pin, changing her role from that of domestic servant to doctor's assistant.

The rules at St Mary's Hospital, formulated in 1849 when the hospital was founded, exemplify the way the ward system worked. The sisters nursed the patients and gave them their medicines. The assistant and night nurses washed the patients, made them clean and comfortable, and reported any sudden or untoward changes in their symptoms to the sister. They cleaned the wards, closets and sculleries, made the beds and could assist the sister in 'nursing the patients *if required*'. A separate team of nurses did the night nursing and stayed on after the day nurses came on duty to help the day staff with making poultices, dressings, breakfasts and washing the bandages and poultice cloths.[3]

The ward system developed first at St Thomas', partly because the wards were large and required two nurses, one of whom had to be in charge. More important was the belief of Miss Sarah Savery, matron from 1816 to 1840, that the sisters'

---

[1]  *BMJ*, 3 January 1880, pp. 11–12.

[2]  See, for example, C. Helmstadter, 'Doctors and Nurses in the London Teaching Hospitals: Class, Gender, Religion and Professional Expertise 1850–90', *Nursing History Review*, 5 (1997): pp. 167–70; M.J. Peterson, *The Medical Profession in Mid-Victorian London* (Berkeley, CA, 1978), pp. 180–87; K. Waddington, 'The Nursing Dispute at Guy's Hospital 1879–1880', *Social History of Medicine*, 8 (1995): pp. 211–30; A. Knight, 'The Great Nursing Dispute of Guy's Hospital 1879–1880', *International History of Nursing Journal*, 3/1 (1997): pp 52–68; J. Moore, *A Zeal for Responsibility: The Struggle for Professional Nursing in Victorian England 1868–83* (Athens, GA, 1988); A. Young, 'Entirely a Woman's Question?', *Journal of Victorian Culture*, 13/1 (2008): pp. 27–35.

[3]  SM/AD/1/2, 6 June 1851 (emphasis added).

work involved so much responsibility that they had to be better-educated and more responsible persons than the working-class assistant nurses from whom the sisters had traditionally been recruited. Savery therefore hired as sisters either women from the shopkeeper class or those who had been head servants in large households. Because these women had no prior hospital experience, Savery made them probationary sisters, supernumeraries who first worked in the matron's office, becoming familiar with the hospital by going on frequent errands into the wards. Next, the probationary sister took charge of a ward where the sister was either off ill or away, and finally, when a vacancy occurred, she was made a ward sister. The length of probation varied depending on how quickly the new sister learnt ward duties and how soon a vacancy occurred. By 1837 there was only one sister at St Thomas' who had been promoted from the ranks of assistant nurse.[4]

## The Spread of the Ward System

In most hospitals, the ward system evolved gradually without a conscious decision on the part of the hospital board, developing at the grassroot level in response to patient and doctor needs, very much as the nurse practitioner movement in the United States developed in the 1960s – on an individual basis in different places.[5] In two hospitals, the Westminster and Middlesex, however, the governors imposed the ward system, thereby giving us records of how the change developed.

*The Westminster 1838*

Distressed by the quality of their nurses, the Westminster governors established a nursing committee in February 1838. After careful investigation of practices at other hospitals, the committee concluded there were two reasons for the Westminster's poor nursing. First, the nurses were underpaid. Second, the hospital had only two types of nurses, day and night nurses, and the night nurses did not report to the day nurses. The solution, the committee proposed, was the ward system. In April the board ruled that, as vacancies occurred, a 'superior class of woman', to be called 'sister', would replace the day nurses. Each sister would be in charge of several wards, supervising and co-ordinating the day and night nurses, keeping good order in her wards and ensuring proper nursing care for the patients day and night. The governors feared that with the possible exception of one or two, none of the 17 nurses then in the hospital would qualify as sisters.[6]

It was not easy to find the superior persons; the new sisters were often guilty of the same misdemeanours as the old nurses. In December 1838 the assistant

---

[4]   LMA/H09/GY/A71/1, p. 673; South, *Facts Relating to Hospital Nurses*, pp. 12–13.

[5]   J. Fairman, *Making Room in the Clinic: Nurse Practitioners and the Evolution of Modern Health Care* (New Brunswick, NJ, 2008), p. 25.

[6]   LMA/H02/WH/A1/31, 3 April 1838.

surgeon reported Sister Ann Smith for several instances of incompetence and gross neglect. She appeared before the board, and was dismissed.[7] In February 1841, John Bicknell, a house visitor,[8] reported that Henry Hoare Ward was in a state of riot and confusion when he visited it the previous Sunday. The sister was unable to control the patients, and the patients refused to tell him the cause of the uproar. One boy said it was not his business to tell who had caused the disturbance, while another just smiled when Bicknell said he would report him to the board. The sister said the riot had arisen over a few potatoes which the matron had sent up. Four patients were mainly responsible, but by the time the House Committee met, three had been discharged, so they could only call in the remaining one to reprimand.[9] In August 1842, another sister, Jane Dawson, was fired for riotous and disorderly behaviour and for refusing to obey the matron's orders as well as threatening to murder Anne Waldron, one of her nurses.[10]

Clinically competent nurses who did not act as 'superior' women were expected to were an especially difficult problem. Mary Anne Taylor, the sister in the female medical wards, was an excellent nurse who was very attentive to her patients, but she had a hasty temper, for which she was reported in January 1844. The board cautioned her. The following December, one of her nurses, Nurse Gillespie, complained that Taylor used abusive and taunting language to her – in fact, such terrible language that Gillespie refused to repeat it. Two board members questioned the patients, who corroborated the nurse's report, but pronounced the sister a good nurse. Taylor was reprimanded again, while Nurse Gillespie was moved to a different ward. It was only in January 1846, when Dr Basham and the secretary complained of Taylor's 'tyrannical, overbearing and bad temper', that she was finally dismissed.[11]

In October 1847 the board learned that Sister Mary Vesey told her patients she always expected a gift, even if it was only a trifle. The mother of Martina Priddis, a child patient in the ward, said that she had given Vesey, among other things, 'several bottles of very acceptable gin', and lace for an apron which the sister requested. The other patients told Priddis that gift giving was the custom, and patients who did not bring presents were not treated well. Susannah Greens, a former patient, said she had given the sister a cap and collar plus a few other trifles. Vesey denied accepting gifts, saying that she paid the patients for the gin and other items. The board told her this behaviour must stop. Vesey was not dismissed until a little over a year later, when a patient complained of her unkindness and harshness, which two surgeons confirmed.[12]

---

[7]   LMA/H02/WH/A1/32, 11 December 1838.

[8]   House visitors were governors whom the board appointed each month to conduct regular inspections of the hospital and to hear patient complaints.

[9]   LMA/H02/WH/A1/32, 2 February 1841.

[10]   LMA/H02/WH/A1/33, 30 August 1842.

[11]   LMA/H02/WH/A1/34, 2 January, 10 December 1844, 13 January 1846.

[12]   LMA/H02/WH/A1/35, 19 October 1847, 23 January 1849.

Inability to keep order, demanding gifts from the patients, and bad tempers and quarrels did not necessarily mean that the sister was an incompetent clinician, and there was such a dearth of able sisters that governors dismissed them with reluctance, and only after previous warnings.

*The Middlesex 1847*

While the doctors pushed to introduce the ward system at the Westminster, at the Middlesex in 1847 the doctors went further and basically took over the nursing. They were, as we have seen, profoundly dissatisfied with Matron Cookesley's nursing service. Since at least 1845 they had been complaining about their nursing service, which they said 'was most inefficient and requires important alteration'.[13] Some nurses were leaving of their own accord, and the old, elderly nurses were dying. Cookesley was dismissing other nurses for all the standard reasons, and in other cases the medical staff was ordering her to discharge nurses for incompetence. Cookesley was finding it almost impossible to find competent replacements.[14]

In 1847 the doctors expressed their distress not only with the inefficiency of the nurses and the high rate of turnover, but also with the understaffing and the nurses' wretched living and working conditions. The nurses did not have regular meals, the night nurses were allowed only six hours out of the 24 for recreation and sleeping, and all were underpaid. The doctors agreed unanimously that many of the nurses were:

> deficient in knowledge of their duty, have frequently been guilty of inebriety and from the constant changes taking place among them have not that interest in the patients and in the good conduct of the wards which better selected nurses with longer service would necessarily entertain.

The nurses' lack of nursing knowledge, the doctors said, placed their patients 'in imminent danger', while order, discipline and cleanliness at the Middlesex were inferior to that in many comparable hospitals.

Of the 31 day, night and assistant nurses, 15 had been in the hospital no more than six months, and 7 no more than three months. In short, only approximately 30 per cent of the nurses had more than six months' experience. The matron did not supervise the nurses adequately, partly because her duties were so onerous, but also because, since she was not a nurse, she simply did not know how. It was absolutely essential, the doctors insisted, that she supervise the nursing care and the nurses' decency of appearance. They had been concerned by the slatternly appearance of their nurses for some time. When they sent their secretary out to investigate the nursing at six other hospitals, he reported that where the ward system was

---

[13]   MH/MBG, 10 June 1845.
[14]   MH/MBG, 4 March, 8 and 22 April, 17 and 29 June, 16 December 1845, 24 February, 8, 22 and 29 December 1846, 12 January and 16 March 1847.

in operation, the head nurses or sisters were enabled to keep a more uniformly neat and cleanly appearance because they were exempted from menial work. The matron should see that nurses did not leave their wards without permission and that they were punctual. The successful treatment of the patients, the doctors stressed, depended primarily on the nurses carrying out medical orders.[15] The result of the doctors' comprehensive complaints was that the governors decided to introduce the ward system. Then, they hoped, a responsible person, the sister, would see that the nurses did their work 'to the satisfaction of the medical officers'.

All the nurses then in the hospital were placed on a 14-day probation, at the end of which, if the doctors did not find them satisfactory, they were to be dismissed. New nurses would undergo the same 14-day probation. The doctors would instruct four to six nurses, selected for their good character and intelligence, while the senior physician and surgeon of the hospital would test the nurses in the delirious wards, where the sickest patients were.

Previously, when nurses took a leave of absence they had to find and pay their own substitute, a standard arrangement in all the hospitals. Under the new rules, the matron, not the nurse, appointed her substitute, and the regular nurse paid only half the substitute's wages while the hospital paid the other half. Furthermore, no nurse on duty could leave her ward for any reason unless directed to so do by the ward's doctor. Nurses could only be absent from the hospital if they had a certificate from one of the senior medical officers. The Medical Committee reported to the Weekly Board at least once a month on the competence of the nurses, their knowledge of their duties and whether they actually performed them. The doctors tried to stop the system of switching nurses from ward to ward: no day or night nurse was to be transferred to another ward or promoted without the written agreement of the doctor of her ward. If a nurse was ill, her substitute was to be found, as far as possible, among the assistant nurses.[16] Since the assistant nurses had virtually no days off, it can only be assumed that they were asked to take on additional wards.

The new sisters were hired in December 1848. The Medical Committee was responsible for their selection and dismissal. The doctors found only one nurse then in the hospital eligible to be a sister and, as at the Westminster, the governors soon discovered there were few respectable and clinically experienced women willing to be sisters.[17]

*St Thomas' 1840s–1850s*

John Flint South, St Thomas' deeply conservative surgeon, passionately supported the ward system and opposed any new-fangled notions of training nurses. His

---

[15]   MH/MBG, 23 February, 17 March, 28 April, 24 August 1847, 6 February 1838.

[16]   Ibid., 24 August 1847, 4 and 18 January 1848.

[17]   Ibid., 19, 26 December 1848; MH/MC, 9 November, 17 December 1850; 2 August 1851; 18 December 1852; 12 March, 12 November 1853.

reaction to the establishment of the Nightingale Fund included the comment in 1857 that the assistant nurses were basically housemaids and needed little instruction 'beyond that of poultice making, enforcement of cleanliness and attention to the patients' wants'.[18] Angered in 1857 by a letter in *The Times* which accused hospital nurses of being inefficient and immoral, he published a pamphlet defending the ward system. This pamphlet presents an idealized picture of the system at St Thomas'. South announced that the Nightingale Fund lacked medical support because there was no need for improved nursing. '*Hospital nursing is well done*,' he proclaimed.[19] He denied the accusations of nurses' immorality. In his 44 years at St Thomas', he claimed he could recall only two instances of immoral misconduct among the sisters, which he thought a lower incidence than among female servants in private families. The sisters, he said, 'bear comparison with a like number of women in any class of society; ... they present continual examples of self-denial and kind solicitude towards the patients'. One sister who had been in South's wards for 17 years had educated one of her two children at King's College Medical School; he was now a member of the Royal College of Surgeons. Another sister, who had been in South's wards for 18 years, had an only child who was now clerk for a respectable builder in the West End of London. There was mutual respect and attachment between the surgeons and sisters, with both surgeons and dressers treating the sisters 'as if they were old superior family servants'.[20] South's identification of the sisters with upper domestic servants was standard.

The probationary period in the matron's office, South explained, ensured the sisters were 'not thrust at once into the wards, ignorant and unfitted for the responsibilities they assume, to pick up a knowledge of their business as they best can'.[21] This was the traditional system which continued for many years in some teaching hospitals.[22] However, the sister's real training, in South's view, came from the physician or surgeon of her ward. He saw her principal duty as taking the doctor's instructions. If the doctor was not interested in teaching her, South said, a sister was likely to make no effort to educate herself and would ultimately 'become more trouble than she was worth'. On the other hand, if the doctor directed and encouraged her and she was reasonably intelligent and interested, she would soon become efficient. South had seen examples of both types of sister, but there was hardly one of his own sisters to whom he was not deeply indebted for the success of many operations and important cases. He stressed the importance of the sisters' assessment skills. Like Dr Golding in 1819, he considered that many patients would have died without the sister's 'untiring watchfulness, disinterestedness, kindness, and large experience of the outbreak of symptoms which require immediate attention'. In acute cases the sister, together

---

[18]   South, *Facts Relating to Hospital Nurses*, p. 16.

[19]   Ibid., pp. 23–4, 30 (original emphasis).

[20]   Ibid., pp. 7–8, 16.

[21]   Ibid., pp. 12–13.

[22]   See, for example, LH/A5/40, 30 November 1880.

with the dresser, was often at the patient's bedside day and night. In those hospitals where operations and bad accidents did best, South said, one could be certain one would find the most attentive and intelligent sisters.[23]

South paid special tribute to Mrs Eliza Roberts, one of his sisters. A specialist in lithotomy and accident cases, she achieved fame during the Crimean War when Florence Nightingale considered her the best of all her hospital nurses. South thought she had more clinical knowledge and experience of hospital matters than anyone else, male or female, in the Crimean War hospitals.[24] Roberts's knowledge and skill in nursing, however, did not extend to the management of her subordinates. In 1848 her ward had the highest turnover among her assistant nurses of any sister in the hospital.

Roberts's problems with her assistant nurses illustrate their unruly, casual nature. Ann Quinn started in October 1847, and was dismissed on 15 January 1848 as not able to do the work. She was followed by Jane Barnard, who started on 22 January and was fired on 17 March for quarrelling with both nurses and patients. Ellen Jarvis started on the same day, but was fired two weeks later on 1 April when Sarah LeFever started. She became ill and had to be warded on 20 May. When LeFever recovered, she did not return to Roberts's ward, but went to the clinical ward, from which she was dismissed the following October for want of sobriety and taking the patients' food. Mary Ann Boyle started on 20 May and was dismissed on 17 June as unable to do the work. Ellen Lowes started on 17 June, but became ill and had to be warded on 23 September. Anne Sweeny started on 30 September and lasted until 2 December, when Mary Ellis replaced her. These seven nurses had an average stay of eight weeks, and the one with the longest stay, Ellen Lowes, was later dismissed for drunkenness. No nurse stayed beyond three months, which was markedly less than the average stay at the Middlesex in 1847, where 30 per cent of the nurses had been in the hospital more than six months. Roberts's night nurse, Sarah Thomas, had been in the ward since June 1839,[25] but as the governors at the Westminster complained in 1838, the night nurses had little to do with the day team.

Eliza Roberts's ward had the highest turnover, but some medical wards were not far behind. In Jacob's Ward, a men's medical ward, Mary Blane came in March 1846, and left without informing the sister on 22 January 1848. She was replaced by Elizabeth Heywood, who left less than a month later, on 19 February, because she could not do the work. Ann Miller replaced her, but left after a month on 25 March because she had been accused of taking money from the patients. Elizabeth Edwards started on 1 April, but after losing several things, left on 11 November, also without telling the sister. Jane Middleton replaced her on 18 November, but a week later was sent to Mary's Ward as a night nurse. Elizabeth Ager took Middleton's place on 25 November, but was sent to Dorcas Ward on 3

---

23  South, *Facts Relating to Hospital Nurses*, pp. 9–10, 15–16.

24  Ibid., pp. 14–15.

25  LMA/H01/ST/C2/1, no pagination; see 'Clinical Ward', 'George Ward'.

March 1849. Middleton was then brought back to Jacob's Ward as a day nurse. By contrast, Margaret Donahue, the night nurse, had been in the ward since 1838.[26]

Mary Hughes illustrates the way assistant and night nurses could take time off, perhaps to spend time with their families, and then return to hospital work. She worked as night nurse in Elizabeth Ward for about a year, leaving on 8 December 1855. Four months later, on 26 April 1856, she returned as a night nurse. Three weeks later she was made day nurse. On 3 January 1857 she left to be married. As Mary Hughes Anderson, she came back as night nurse in the casualty ward on 24 July 1858, leaving on 8 January 1859. She returned two months later, again as a night nurse, on 5 March, leaving a little over a month later, on 16 April 1859.[27]'Two of the six nurses in Jacob's Ward remained in the system, providing another illustration of the way nurses were switched from ward to ward, but where did the other four go? Did they apply to another hospital, did they take up domiciliary nursing, were they just taking time off, as Mary Hughes seems to have done, or did they find some other means of livelihood? We do not know, for hospitals did not keep records of these women until much later in the century. The Matron's Register at St Thomas' for 1848 and part of 1849 in which we found this information is one of only two records which take cognizance of assistant and night nurses in the earlier part of the century that we have been able to locate.

The assistant nurses were almost on the lowest rung on the nursing ladder, and for this reason, as well as their peripatetic work habits, we know little about them as individuals. The only contemporary detailed description of an assistant nurse which we have found comes from Miss Fowler, a visitor to St Thomas' in 1853. She described the 'harsh' or 'unkind' treatment frequently mentioned in hospital minute books but almost never detailed. Fowler had gone to the hospital with her friend Milly, who was taking clean linen to her husband who had had his leg amputated. They were met inside the door of the ward by an assistant nurse, an old woman wearing a dirty black net cap, a plaid cross-over shawl over her shoulders and a blue and white checked apron. Her dress had once been black, but was green and brown from wear, and Fowler wondered when she had last washed her face.

A patient called 'Nurse', and the nurse went over to a man who looked terribly ill. She leaned over him to hear what he had to say, and then pulled him upright, shook him, smacked his head soundly and then pushed him down on his pillow and threw the sheet over him. Milly's husband swore, and said that if he had both his legs he would like to kick the old devil for the way she laid into that poor dying chap. Milly asked him if the nurse laid into him in the same way. He replied:

> If she did I should forget she was a woman and give her one she would not forget. Look here, Milly, when you go out she will come carrying after you expecting you to give her some money. If you do you will hear of it when I get home.

26    Ibid., 'Jacob's Ward'.
27    Ibid., insert.

Milly's husband was quite right. The nurse followed Miss Fowler and Milly down the ward, wrinkling up her dirty old face as she asked, 'A tizzie, a tizzie for a nurse.'[28] Milly gave her the 6d.[29] Where was the sister of the ward? Did her assistant nurse behave in this manner when the sister was there? Not all the ward system's sisters were watchful and kind.

There were, of course, exceptions to the high rate of turnover among the assistant nurses. Jane Davis was a sister in a male venereal ward from 1831, and sister of the cholera ward in 1849. Despite the strenuous nursing in these wards, she was an exception both in her length of stay and in her gift for working with her subordinates. In 1849 she received a 10 guinea gratuity for 'the zeal and perseverance with which she carried out her arduous duties during the [cholera] epidemic'. She continued to work 'with the greatest cheerfulness, kindness and ability' until her health collapsed, forcing her to retire in 1854. Davis's night nurse, Ellen Jones, started in October 1825, and by 1849 was the longest-staying nurse in the hospital. Davis's day nurse, Ann Green, had worked with her since June 1839, and was the longest-staying day nurse. Green may well have gone with Davis to the cholera ward, for she died of cholera in 1849.[30]

Under the ward system, the sisters tended to stay for considerable lengths of time, especially on the less demanding services, and some became highly competent. The sisters of the female surgical wards at St Thomas' stayed an average of eight years in 1848. In the men's medical wards they stayed almost as long, an average of seven years, but on women's medical wards, traditionally a heavy service, the average was only one year. Many night nurses also remained in the hospital for some years,[31] but they did not benefit from their longer experience because they were so isolated. The assistant nurses were essentially a casual workforce. With very poor general educations, no training in nursing, little or no support from their superiors, and poor living and working conditions, it was extremely difficult for assistant and night nurses to become effective nurses. It was not surprising that so many left or were dismissed because they were 'unable to do the work'.

## The Intensified Need for Clinical Experience

The introduction of anaesthesia, first used in London in December 1846, had a profound influence on the need for clinically experienced nurses, or what the hospital community was coming to call 'skilled nursing'. At first, anaesthesia was used selectively, and the number and length of operations did not increase

---

[28]   'Tizzie' was slang for a sixpenny piece.

[29]   LMA/H01/ST/Y4.

[30]   LMA/H01/ST/A8/2, 25 September 1849; LMA/H01/ST/A6/13, 14 November 1854; LMA/H01/ST/C2/1, Naples Ward.

[31]   LMA/H01/ST/C2/1, passim.

significantly for several years.[32] By contrast, the impact on nursing services was dramatic and almost immediate. It was no coincidence that the Middlesex took action to reform its nursing in 1847. Post-anaesthetic care intensified the constantly growing need for more skilled nursing. This was especially true at night, when the night watchers, the weakest link in the nursing service, were in charge. All the teaching hospitals began hiring more day and night nurses to meet this need. Usually, they were extra – or what we now call 'casual' – nurses. At University College Hospital in April 1853 the board was paying £21 17s. per week for extra nurses, which amounted to nearly half the total cost of all the regular day and night nurses.[33] The upgrading of the night nursing following the introduction of anaesthesia is striking: the London in 1847, St George's in 1849, University College in 1851 and St Thomas' in 1854 all made significant efforts to improve their night nursing.

In December 1849 a large number of assistant nurses at the London Hospital were off sick. Two wards had regular night nurses who worked that shift exclusively, but in all the other wards the day nurses covered nights, leaving their wards at 5 p.m. instead of 10 p.m. so they could have four or five hours of rest before starting the night shift at 9.30 or 10 p.m. Then they had to work their normal day shift the next day. The nurses therefore worked 13–13½ hours the first day and 22 hours the second.[34] The apothecary thought excessive fatigue was causing the nurses' illnesses, and urged the governors to hire more permanent night nurses. It was unfair to both nurses and patients, he said, to expect the nurses to work such long hours. The governors agreed to hire 14 new night nurses. Matron Jane Nelson insisted that she had to pay them a premium to secure what she termed 'respectable, intelligent women'.[35]

At University College Hospital in April 1851 a medical student sent the governors a £50 donation he had secured from Samuel Gurney, the wealthy Quaker banker and philanthropist. Gurney was the brother of prison reformer Elizabeth Fry, who, as we will see in the next chapter, was also interested in nursing. The £50 was for an additional night nurse in the male accident wards for two years. The following May, Gurney donated another £50 for two more night nurses in the same wards. The medical student was Joseph Lister, soon to become famous for his antiseptic practice. Lister himself donated another £50 for more nurses the following year.[36]

The sisters at the Westminster do not appear to have successfully co-ordinated the day and night teams as the governors had hoped in 1838, because in 1853 the

[32]   F.F. Cartwright, *The Development of Modern Surgery* (London, 1967), pp. 35–6.

[33]   UCH/A1/2/1, 27 April 1853.

[34]   See, for example, Yeo, *Nursing at Bart's*, p. 25; A. Terton, *Lights and Shadows in a Hospital* (London, 1902), pp. 11–15. Terton does not name the London teaching hospital in which she worked, but internal evidence indicates it was the Middlesex.

[35]   LH/A4/10, 1 December 1847.

[36]   UCH/A1/2/1, 9 April, 21 May 1851, 7 July 1852.

Medical Committee again addressed this issue. The doctors wanted to use the same nurses at night as in the day, first to establish more continuity of care, and second because the day nurses were more competent than the night watchers. The hospital began rotating the assistant nurses onto nights every other week. To make the night duty more palatable, the governors gave the nurses new privileges when on night duty: when they finished cleaning the wards, they could, with the matron's consent, go out for an hour, returning before noon to help with the patients' meals. They could then sleep from 2 p.m. until 9.30 p.m. and go on duty at 10 p.m.[37]

St Thomas' and St Bartholomew's had had regular night watchers since at least the eighteenth century. In the 1840s, St Thomas' began insisting that all nurses live in the hospital; John Flint South remarked on the improvement in the nursing, especially the night nursing, resulting from this policy.[38] When the nurses did not appear for work, as often happened, their superiors could simply go to their dormitory and roust them out of bed. In 1854 the St Thomas' governors changed the matron's job description to include occasional visits to the female wards in the evening to see that the sisters were not sleeping outside the hospital and the nurses were not away from their wards without the matron's permission.[39]

It was at St George's Hospital where, after a number of false starts, the first partially successful steps in securing co-ordination between the day and night nurses took place. In 1849 the governors gave the night nurses the same wage as the head nurses and removed their cleaning duties because, they said, they interfered with their more important nursing duties. Under the old system the medical officers rarely or never saw the night nurses. Now the night nurses would come on duty an hour earlier, at 9 p.m., so that the day nurses and the medical officers could give them the necessary instructions and directions for their patients. The head nurses were ordered to teach the night nurses how to carry out medical orders – another indication that the old night watchers did not have basic nursing skills. Four of the 11 night nurses then in the hospital were unable to perform their new duties.[40] In November 1852 the hospital introduced another improvement in the night nurses' working conditions: the matron hired a supernumerary nurse who would take the duty of each night nurse for one night every 24 days so that each nurse could have a day off.[41]

After a four-year trial of the new system of treating the night nurses on a par with the head nurses, it would appear that the new night nurses were not up to the increased responsibility. As at the Westminster, the hospital decided to do away with the separate team of night nurses. As the old night nurses left, assistant nurses took their position with a small increase in salary. A number of the night nurses

---

[37]  LMA/H02/WH/A1/36, 18 January, 1 February, 15 and 29 March 1853.

[38]  South, *Facts Relating to Hospital Nurses*, p. 17.

[39]  LMA/H01/ST/A6/12, 27 December 1853. The steward was responsible for discipline in the male wards.

[40]  SGH/MBG, 22 August, 26 September, 14 November 1849.

[41]  Ibid., 24 November, 29 December 1852.

were discharged, and all vacancies among the head nurses were to be filled by experienced night nurses. This system does not appear to have worked either, for in 1853 the hospital decided to create the position of night superintendent. This new position carried a salary of £70 a year, which it was hoped would ensure the services of a superior nurse.[42] The salary compared very favourably with those of the other nurses. St George's paid the head nurses £20–£31 10s. a year, and the experienced matron £100. When a new matron was hired in 1855, she was paid £70.[43]

Harriet Richardson, the new night superintendent of St George's and the first such officer in the teaching hospitals, started work in September 1853. Her salary was raised to £80 in December, suggesting that she had made considerable improvements.[44] However, she was not a nurse. 'At one time,' Miss Eva Lückes, matron of the London Hospital, wrote 33 years later, 'any trustworthy person was considered competent to walk through a hospital as night superintendent, the chief duty attached to her appointment being to see that the nurses were awake and apparently attending to their duties' rather than wandering about the building.[45] This was essentially what Richardson did, for in December 1855, when the night nurse in Princess Ward failed to call the house surgeon to see a critically ill post-operative child, it was noted that Richardson had not visited the ward. She explained that there was no system in place to keep her informed of critical cases. One of the doctors then ordered the head nurse in each ward to give Richardson in person and in writing the names and numbers of the beds of patients requiring special attention. In addition, Richardson was to accompany the apothecary and house surgeon on their rounds at 9 p.m.[46]

When Richardson resigned in 1857, the board specified that the new night superintendent must not only be highly respectable, but must thoroughly understand nursing duties because she had to supervise the entire nursing of the hospital during the night.[47] Nursing knowledge was finally acknowledged to be as important as respectability, but it seemed impossible to find a respectable nurse who was willing to work nights. Miss Mullock came for two months, but was found unsuitable. Miss Green was then kept on trial for nearly three months, but was found incompetent because she had no nursing experience. The matron and apothecary then recommended Elizabeth Johnston, the head nurse of Burton Ward. She was appointed at a proposed salary of £80, but apparently the board thought

42     Ibid., 16 March, 9 April, 14 December 1853.
43     Ibid., 16 February, 23 March 1853, 26 September 1855.
44     Ibid., 14 September, 14 December 1853.
45     E.C.E. Lückes, *Hospital Sisters and their Duties* (London, 1886), p. 176.
46     SGH/MBG, 5 and 12 December 1855.
47     SGH/Minutes of Committee to Elect a Night Superintendent, Miscellaneous Committee Book 1857–60, 17 June 1857.

it was too much money for someone who was not a lady, for in the end she was paid £40.[48]

Despite the clinically experienced night superintendent, the co-ordination between day and night staff remained unsatisfactory. The night nurses were, with a few exceptions, inefficient and insubordinate, and the high rate of turnover and traditional 'irregularities' continued. The governors thought Johnston did not control her staff; she complained that the matron did not support her when she reported night nurses for dereliction of duty. In 1864 the governors finally gave Johnston the same authority over the night nurses as a head nurse had over her assistant nurses. Her 'long, valuable and laborious services' were rewarded with an increase in salary of £1 a year to a maximum of £50. Her hours were shortened and she was allowed to leave the hospital for two hours a day. Johnston's new job description in 1864 indicates that many problems at the beginning of the century persisted: Johnston was to see that the night nurses looked after those patients who could not look after themselves, that medicines were properly administered, and that the nurses were not extracting gifts from the patients. Johnston did not enjoy her increased salary and two free hours a day for long, because she died less than a year later.[49]

### Increasing Unacceptability of Nurses' Working and Living Conditions

Working and living conditions for nurses, particularly in the newer and less wealthy hospitals, were extremely harsh. In an effort to counteract the enormous difficulties in recruiting and retaining respectable nurses, hospitals began, as we have seen, to improve the nurses' hours and lighten their duties. In 1851, Dr Lionel Beale, who had just finished his six-month term as physician's assistant at King's College Hospital, sent the Committee of Management a long letter explaining that so much hard physical labour was demanded of the nurses that they could not give reasonable care to their patients. For 15 hours out of the 24 each nurse administered medicines, dressed wounds and so on. She also had to scrub down the centre of her ward every morning, and twice a week scour the whole ward, moving every bed, which took about three hours, during which time the nurse was unable to give her patients the care which, Beale said, was such an important part of the successful treatment of disease. The nurses usually managed to carry out their orders but only at the expense of their health. During Beale's six months, five of the eight day nurses had been off sick due to overwork.

Beale suggested that the hospital hire scrubbers to relieve the nurses of some of their duties. He thought it essential to hire extra night nurses for the critical cases. Many night nurses had worked all day, and were so tired they were physically unable to give the unremitting attention which these patients required. The women

[48] Ibid., 26 August, 21 November 1857; SGH/MBG, 27 April 1864.
[49] SGH/MBG, 27 January, 3 February, 27 April 1864, 8 February 1865.

were paid only 1s. a night (£18 5s. a year) and given no food or drink. At the same time, their patients were sometimes ordered as much as a half pint of brandy, beef tea, arrowroot and other nourishments, which the hungry nurses often consumed themselves. Beale suggested paying them a little more plus giving them some beer, as did other hospitals.

The committee hired four charwomen to do the scouring, shortened the night nurses' tour of duty to 14½ hours and agreed to pay the extra night nurses 1s. 3d. a night. They relieved the day nurses of all the scrubbing, assigning this duty to the night nurses, gave the day nurses a little time off – from the time the patients went to bed until 10 p.m. *if* there were no urgent cases in the ward and *if* there was a nurse on every floor. To stop the nurses from doing their personal washing in the wards, the hospital agreed to pay to send their laundry out.[50] As in all the teaching hospitals, the new policy resulted in a major increase in the female staff. In 1843 the staff at King's College Hospital consisted of nine nurses; by 1854 there were ten day nurses, four night nurses and one extra nurse plus ten scrubbers, a total of 24 regular and one extra staff.[51]

In the 1850s the Westminster began giving time off for vacations, and by the 1860s was paying the substitutes for nurses who were ill. This was the policy at St Mary's, St Bartholomew's, the London, University College, the Middlesex and St George's Hospitals. In March 1860 the Westminster raised the wages of all the nurses, and in 1864 started giving the sisters three weeks and nurses two weeks a year of paid holiday.[52] In this, nursing was ahead of other occupations – perhaps a recognition of its wearing nature. Until the twentieth century, paid holidays were rare for manual workers, as nurses were then considered. *Unpaid* week-long breaks first began to make their appearance among textile workers, generally considered better-paid female labour, only in the late 1870s and 1880s.[53]

The wretched accommodation hospitals gave their nurses remained a problem with which hospitals would struggle for many years to come. At mid-century, hospitals provided only sleeping space for the nurses; there were no dining or common rooms for them. As more nurses became necessary, finding decent space in buildings which had been built for much smaller nursing staffs became an almost insoluble problem. Yet hospital administrators were anxious to have their staffs living in, in order to facilitate discipline and ensure they showed up for work. When the Middlesex reformed its nursing in 1847–48, the hospital made it a rule that the nurses were 'to be kept as much as possible within the hospital' to give the matron better control over them. The board wanted the night nurses, who had traditionally lived outside the hospital, to sleep in the house, but had no proper place to put them. When the hospital hired five additional nurses in 1848, three were crammed into

---

[50]   KH/CM/M4, 23 May 1851.

[51]   KH/CM/M2, 5 April & 9 May 1843; KH/CM/M4, 27 January 1854.

[52]   LMA/H02/WH/A1/37, 3 October 1854; WH/A1/40, 1 July 1862; WH/A1/41, 19 July & 4 October 1864.

[53]   Hoppen, *The Mid-Victorian Generation*, p. 367.

the day nurses' dormitory while two slept in the bathrooms of their wards. In an effort to give each nurse some privacy, the hospital installed partitions in the nurses' dormitory, but until they were able to provide better sleeping quarters, the Weekly Board said, it was impossible to further improve the nursing.[54]

In 1849, St Thomas' built two new dormitories for the nurses on the upper floor of the new, rebuilt north wing. Each dormitory had two fireplaces, there was a kitchen and scullery attached with hot water, and hot water in the nurses' lavatories as well. Each sister had a bedroom and a sitting room, both with a fireplace.[55] These were more comfortable arrangements than in the older parts of the hospital, and far superior to those at any of the other hospitals, including the other two endowed hospitals. The situation at Guy's was more typical. As in most hospitals, there were a number of different dormitories for the nurses, squeezed in where the authorities could find space. In 1855, two years after Dr Steele came to Guy's as professional administrator, he rearranged the nurses' housing, converting the surgeons' out-patient waiting rooms in Guy's House, the original building, into a dormitory for the nurses and helpers. He installed an 'overlooker' in an apartment at the entrance to the dormitory so that she could maintain order and see that the nurses reported on time for work.[56] The dormitory was so wet, however, that the damp damaged the nurses' clothes. They asked for some additional means of heating; Steele gave them hot water bottles. They were still complaining of the damp and cold 20 years later.[57] There were rats in one basement dormitory, and Sister Clinical asked many times for some means of stopping the disturbances to the nurses in the Hunt's House dormitory. Steele thought a door at the entrance to the dormitory would solve the problem. However, even with the door in place, occasional irregularities arose from friends of the patients going into the dormitory. Steele put a sign which said 'Private' on the door.[58]

At St Bartholomew's the sisters lived in one room which had been partitioned off the staircase landing. They had formerly slept in a dormitory in another part of the building, but at the end of the eighteenth century,[59] when the new medicine started making 24-hour nursing care and observation necessary, these rooms were constructed so the sisters could be immediately adjacent to the ward and on call 24 hours a day. The new rooms had a window, but no fireplace. In the double wards, so called because there was a door between the two wards and one sister supervised both, the nurses slept in a tiny room also carved out of the stair landing.

[54] MH/MBG, 18 and 25 January, 3 February 1848.

[55] LMA/H01/ST/A6/12, 9 January 1849; LMA/H01/ST/A/114/016.

[56] LMA/H09/GY/A3/8/1, 7 March 1855.

[57] LMA/H09/GY/A67/2/1, 16 November, 16 May 1860; LMA/H09/GY/A67/3, 23 January 1867; LMA/H09/GY/A67/5, 17 January 1877.

[58] LMA/H09/GY/A67/2/1, 25 July and 12 September 1860; LMA/H09/GY/A67/2/3, 16 April 1862.

[59] Moore, *The History of St Bartholomew's Hospital*, vol. 2, pp. 759–60.

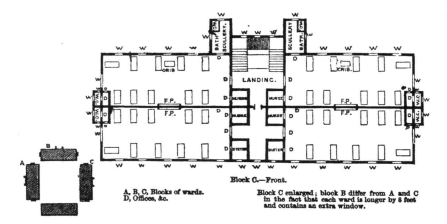

Figure 3.1     Floor plan of double wards at St Bartholomew's Hospital, *c.* 1860. Bathrooms and water closets had been added to the eighteenth-century building. Each four windowless nurses' rooms had two beds shared by three nurses. The night nurse used a day nurse's bed.

*Note*s: Key: D = door; W = window; FP = fireplace.

*Source: PP*, 1864, vol. 28, p. 571.

St George's was completely rebuilt in the early 1830s, when it seemed that a much smaller number of nurses was needed than was the case by the 1860s. When the hospital hired the night superintendent, she was forced to live out because there was no suitable space for a 'respectable person' in the hospital. In 1857, 47 nurses slept in 21 rooms. Of these rooms, eight had chimneys but three had no grate, and 13 had no chimney at all. Two rooms, which housed eight women, had neither fireplaces nor windows. The night nurses had nowhere to cook their meals except the small, airless rooms in which they slept. The normal requirement per person was generally considered 1,000 cubic feet of air, but none of the 21 rooms met this standard. Only one head nurse had a sleeping room to herself. Nor did the hospital supply coal to those nurses who had fireplaces in their rooms. The chimneys were used purely for ventilation.[60]

The doctors at Charing Cross Hospital repeatedly complained that it was understaffed and the nurses inefficient. Increases in the nurses' wages had failed to attract a better class of woman. In 1863 the governors reached the same conclusion as had the governors at the Middlesex in 1848 – it was simply not possible to attract respectable nurses until they could offer better accommodation. The governors noted that the Nightingale Training School and the Anglican Sisters at University College and King's College Hospitals provided superior

---

[60]     SGH/MBG, 1 and 16 December 1858.

nursing with great benefit to the patients, but those hospitals also provided better accommodation for their nurses. At Charing Cross, there simply was not enough space in the building to house nurses comfortably.[61] Overcrowded accommodation was one of the outstanding characteristics of the life of the poor.[62] In the earlier part of the nineteenth century, skilled – as opposed to ordinary – workers in one of the better-paid trades usually lived with their whole families in a single furnished room. The radical organizer Francis Place, a successful tailor, advised artisans to try to maintain two rooms, one for domestic use and one for a workshop. Only the aristocrats of labour could hope to occupy three or four rooms.[63] Sanitarians who went into working-class homes in the 1860s were horrified by the conditions under which these families lived. Twenty, 30 or sometimes 40 persons lived in houses built for a single family, or at most two families. Both children and adults were obliged 'To live, sleep, and perform the offices of nature in the same room … and it may be with other relatives, or possibly with strangers'.[64]

Still, even if working-class women were used to much worse living conditions, arrangements such as those at the Middlesex or St George's were hardly a draw for respectable, competent women. The standard of living was rising, and able persons of any class would not accept a nurse's position if they had to live in such squalid quarters.

## The Ward System Assessed

How well did the ward system work? Many doctors and lay governors were dissatisfied with it and with the ward sisters who were its lynchpin. In 1843 the governors at King's College Hospital were experiencing a financial crisis and decided to dismiss all their sisters. Their initial motive was to save money, but they were also dissatisfied with the sisters. They did not nurse the patients themselves, but rather delegated their duties to the assistant nurses. They also relied on the assistant nurses for information about the patients, creating what the doctors considered a very dangerous situation.[65] The St Thomas' sisters impressed John Flint South and the Charity Commissioners, but their governors were less pleased. In 1843, in the hope of attracting 'a better class of person', they significantly increased the sisters' base salaries.[66] Two years later they raised the wages of the assistant nurses. In 1855 the hospital cut expenditures on drugs and decreased the wages of the medical officers and servants, but was afraid to cut the nurses' wages.[67]

[61]   CCH/MBG, 7 January 1863, 28 February 1867.

[62]   G. Best, *Mid-Victorian Britain 1851–75* (London, 1971), pp. 58–60.

[63]   Rule, *The Labouring Classes in Early Industrial England*, pp. 87–90, 94, 98.

[64]   J. Hollingshead, *Ragged London in 1861* (London, 1861), p. 256.

[65]   KH/CM/M2, 5 April, 9 May 1843.

[66]   LMA/H01/ST/A1/8, 22 November 1843.

[67]   LMA/H01/ST/A1/6/13, 9 January 1855.

In 1858 the governors decided, like the King's College Hospital governors, that the sisters delegated too many of their duties to the assistant nurses. They were even unhappier with the assistant nurses, whom they considered 'undesirable people' to be attending patients,[68] an opinion which Miss Fowler's observations support.

Writing in 1884, Dr J.S. Bristowe characterized the old sisters at St Thomas' as unimpressive. When he entered the hospital as a medical student in 1846, he thought the sisters respectable, but only two or three really efficient. Those two or three were some of the most able and intelligent women he had ever met, but, he said, they were exceptions.[69] Bristowe may well have been judging the sisters in the 1840s with standards of the 1880s, but even so, it would seem that his judgement that the highly competent sisters in the 1840s were exceptions is a fair one. In 1859, Richard Whitfield, the resident medical officer at St Thomas', described Mrs Eliza Roberts in the same way, as an exception. She was, he said, 'one in a century of thousands, a thorough practical nurse'.[70]

The ward system recognized the sisters' need for nursing expertise, and the improvements which all the hospitals made in working and living conditions were a major step forward. However, the system had serious failings. First, its highly decentralized nature hinged on the *voluntary* efforts of two individuals: the doctor and the sister of the ward. Many doctors gave scant attention to their hospital patients and did not teach their sisters,[71] while some sisters were not interested in learning – something which even South admitted. Second, the fine practical education which some doctors gave their sisters did not filter down to the assistant nurses: few sisters made any effort to teach their staff. Even when the sisters were willing, the very casual, unstable nature of the nursing workforce, as well as the way nurses were constantly switched from one ward to another, made systematic instruction almost impossible. Yet the ward system developed exactly when nursing had become so much more labour-intensive and demanding of professional judgement that it was impossible for one person, the sister, to do all the skilled nursing. One person could not carry out the expert 24-hour assessment and care of patients which the new medicine demanded. The lack of co-ordination between the night and the day staff, so destructive of good patient care, was a third major failing. Even at St George's, with experienced Head Nurse Johnston as night

---

[68]  LMA/H01/ST/A1/9, 25 May 1858.

[69]  J.S. Bristowe, 'How Far Should our Hospitals be Training Schools for Nurses?' (1884), BL/Cup.401.i.7.(8.), pp. 9–10.

[70]  BL 47742, fols 65–6.

[71]  R.C. Lucas, 'In Memorium – Walter Moxon, MD', *Guy's Hospital Reports*, XLIV (1887): p. 16: 'His hospital patients were treated with almost paternal care, and he was most imperative in his instructions to the nurses, never allowing any chance of possible neglect.' cf. S. Wilks, 'In Memorium George Owen Rees, M.D., F.R.S', *Guy's Hospital Reports*, XLVI (1889): pp. xxxi–xxxii :'Rees had an 'aversion to low and ignorant persons …. After seeing his private patients at home, he would proceed to the hospital, where he … was probably too rapid in his rounds to give much time to his cases.'

superintendent, many old problems persisted, in part because, like the old matrons, Johnston had inadequate authority to carry out her mission.

The ward system did give those doctors who were interested in the nursing control over the sister of their wards.[72] When the newer central and training school systems were introduced later in the century, it was this control of the nursing in their own wards which the doctors at Guy's, and other teaching hospitals, would fight so fiercely to preserve.

---

[72] *BMJ*, 17 January 1880, p. 90.

# Chapter 4
# Early Efforts at Training

Some hospital wards ran well under the ward system, but much remained to be done to bring the assistant and night nurses up to an acceptable clinical standard. The same was true of many sisters. In addition, as the reformation of manners took hold, there was the whole issue of Victorian standards of propriety and respectability, which only some sisters and fewer nurses met. In this chapter we first explore overseas influences on nurse training in England. We explain why Roman Catholic[1] models of nursing had little impact on early attempts to provide structured training for nurses. In contrast, the Deaconess Institute at Kaiserswerth, Germany, a highly successful institution which trained large numbers of nurses who met the requirements of Victorian respectability, was profoundly influential. The Kaiserswerth Institute directly influenced two early efforts to provide training for English nurses: Elizabeth Fry's nursing institution founded in 1840, and Florence Nightingale's reorganization of the Hospital for Gentlewomen at Harley Street in 1853–54.

## Catholic Sisters: The Impact of Political Restrictions

There were a number of expert, highly respectable nurses in England in the 1840s and 1850s: Catholic religious nurses who came from the Continent and Ireland. As historian Sioban Nelson has demonstrated, in the early nineteenth century they were the only nurses generally considered respectable.[2] While convents and monasteries had been dissolved in England during the Reformation, they had, of course, continued on the Continent and elsewhere. In the first part of the nineteenth century there was a resurgence of sisterhoods, notably in France and Belgium. Taking an international and evangelical outlook, these new Catholic sisterhoods founded convents in many foreign countries. In 1829, the passing of the Catholic Relief Act (Catholic Emancipation) permitted the establishment of Catholic convents in England. The first was established in London in 1830; by 1850 there were 51 in England, and by 1860, 118. The vast majority belonged to active orders, and some provided nursing services.[3]

---

[1]  Following common usage, hereafter termed 'Catholic'.
[2]  Nelson, *Say Little, Do Much*, p. 163.
[3]  S. O'Brien, 'French Nuns in Nineteenth Century England', *Past and Present*, 154 (1997): pp. 144–5, 152, 154, 159.

The Irish sisterhoods also established many convents throughout the world. Of particular interest from a nursing viewpoint were the Sisters of Mercy, who in 1839 sent one of their most competent mother superiors, Mary Clare Moore, to organize a convent in Bermondsey, London. Moore was highly successful, and personally founded eight other autonomous Mercy convents in England, ranging geographically from the south coast to Yorkshire. Among their many ministries, the Bermondsey nuns nursed the sick poor in their homes, and most famously, sent eight Sisters to join Nightingale during the Crimean War.[4]

The sisterhoods' centralized structure worked well for teaching nursing, which the Sisters did very competently, using the concept of probation – a largely apprenticeship model. Yet, notwithstanding their highly skilled practice, these Sisters had little impact on hospital nursing in England.[5] Despite the many converts they made,[6] their work was primarily among Irish immigrants. More importantly, residual political restrictions on Catholics meant they could not nurse in any of the prestigious teaching hospitals. Of equal consequence, the presence of Catholic sisters – and by 1848 there were 16 convents in London alone – incited the vicious anti-Catholicism which pervaded all classes of English society. Many English Protestants identified the Pope with the Antichrist and Catholicism with the Scarlet Woman of the book of Revelation;[7] for these people, the sisterhoods were sinister devices of Rome. English anti-Catholicism meant, as Nelson wrote, that nursing reform in England had to be a Protestant endeavour.[8]

## Kaiserswerth Diakoniewerk: A Protestant and Genteel Training[9]

The Diakoniewerk in Kaiserswerth, a small town near Düsseldorf in Germany, profoundly influenced early nursing reform in England. This deaconess training institute consisted of an orphanage, schools, an asylum for female ex-prisoners, and a hospital. It was established in 1836 by Theodor Fliedner, a Lutheran pastor.[10] The drive, vision and independent spirit of Friederike Fliedner, Theodor's first wife, established the form and tone of the Diakoniewerk Institution. She had been brought up in the Reformed Church, which was organized more as a democratic

[4]    M.C. Sullivan (ed.), *The Friendship of Florence Nightingale and Mary Clare Moore* (Philadelphia, PA, 1999), pp. 5, 8.

[5]    Nelson, *Say Little, Do Much*, p. 64.

[6]    See BA, passim 1839–54.

[7]    O. Chadwick, *The Victorian Church* (2 vols, 3rd edn, London, 1971), vol. 1, pp. 287, 505–8; W.L. Arnstein, *Protestant vs. Catholic in Mid-Victorian England: Mr. Newdegate and the Nuns* (Columbia, MO, 1982), pp. 3–4.

[8]    Nelson, *Say Little, Do Much*, p. 78.

[9]    This section was written by Joyce Schroeder MacQueen.

[10]    Florence Nightingale, *The Institution of Kaiserswerth on the Rhine* (London, 1851), p. 11.

community based on the individual's responsibility under God rather than as a religious hierarchy. Thus, the Kaiserswerth deaconesses formed a council that governed their own affairs. Friederike Fliedner is celebrated as having actively assisted nursing 'in establishing its independence with regards to doctors, the clergy, governing bodies and authorities'.[11] In 1841, for example, she insisted on travelling with four deaconesses to their new assignment even though three of her children were severely ill and her husband barely convalescing. When she arrived home, one of her children had died, followed a few days later by another. Her long letter home describing the terrible conditions of the hospital where the nurse deaconesses were to be placed explains the need for her journey. Friederike Fliedner met with the whole committee of hospital directors and informed them that 'if conditions are not altered we will not allow the Sisters to stay'.[12] By contrast, ladies in England could not speak directly to hospital committees. This convention applied even to a lady of Florence Nightingale's eminence. When the Nightingale School was established, all her dealings with the St Thomas' Hospital board were through the men who headed the Nightingale Fund Council.

When Friederike died in 1842, Theodor Fliedner quickly remarried. Caroline Bertheau, his second wife, had been director of nursing at Hamburg's General Hospital. In Kaiserswerth she became known as Mother Fliedner, directing the deaconess and nursing programmes, as well as being stepmother to five children and eventually bearing eight children herself.[13] Like her predecessor, Caroline took charge of nursing and nursing training at Kaiserswerth. The success of Kaiserswerth meant that this was no small matter: in 1851 there were 90 deaconesses; by 1864 there were 400.[14]

A number of foreign women trained for short periods at Kaiserswerth, helping to spread its influence internationally. Among them were some of the first generation of British nursing leaders, including Agnes Jones, Florence Lees and Lucy Osburn.[15] As explored below, Elizabeth Fry was profoundly inspired by a visit in 1840. Elizabeth Ferard, who became the first deaconess within the Anglican Church, spent time training at Kaiserswerth and subsequently offered charitable nursing services in London.[16] The best-known visitor was Florence Nightingale.

[11]   D.A. Sticker, *Theodor Fliedner and Nursing* (Düsseldorf, 1972), p. 7.

[12]   M.A. Nutting and L.L. Dock, *A History of Nursing* (4 vols, New York, [1907], 1935), vol. 2, p. 22, citing translated letter from Friederike Fliedner.

[13]   Sticker, *Theodor Fliedner and Nursing*, p. 8; Nutting and Dock, *A History of Nursing*, p. 25.

[14]   WI/Ms 9025/24/7; LMA/H1/ST/NC1/64/21.2.

[15]   J.C. Ross and J. Ross, *A Gifted Touch: A Biography of Agnes Jones* (Worthing, West Sussex, 1988), pp. 13–14; M. Baly, *A History of the Queen's Nursing Institute, 100 Years 1887–1987* (London, 1987), pp. 12–13; J. Godden, *Lucy Osburn, a Lady Displaced: Florence Nightingale's Envoy to Australia* (Sydney, 2006), pp. 29–30.

[16]   V. Bonham, 'Ferard, Elizabeth Catherine (1825–1883)', *Oxford Dictionary of National Biography*, <http://www.oxforddnb.com/view/article/39512> (accessed 10 July

She spent two weeks there in 1850, following which, at the instigation of Theodor Fliedner, she wrote the booklet *The Institution of Kaiserswerth on the Rhine*. A year later, she returned for three months' training. Although she later decried its quality of nursing, she incorporated aspects of the Kaiserswerth system into her work at the Harley Street hospital and the Nightingale School of Nursing at St Thomas' Hospital. Like the London teaching hospitals, Kaiserswerth Diakoniewerk was a charitable institution which relied on donations. Its income was supplemented by the fees paid by visitors and payment from those patients who could afford it. The institution attempted to be as self-sufficient as possible, and the deaconesses lived a frugal life.[17] As in Catholic sisterhoods, the deaconesses completed a probationary period, and after training, could be sent to missions elsewhere in the country or abroad.[18] The radical aspect of Kaiserswerth was that all the deaconesses, and visitors, lived and worked together regardless of class. Working with individuals from a variety of social classes was a formative experience for many women, including Florence Nightingale, who later supported the same principle at St Thomas' Hospital.[19]

Service to God through charitable work was the dominating focus at Kaiserswerth. The crux of Florence Nightingale's many criticisms of Kaiserswerth as a nurse training centre was that treating the sick was a secondary concern. By the mid-nineteenth century its hospital had 100 beds, with separate wards for men, women and children. Patients were admitted with the usual range of medical conditions, such as scrofula, scabies, croup, fever and tuberculosis, but there was little surgery. Despite being deeply religious, Nightingale was distressed that at Kaiserswerth 'the religious principle over-ruled everything – even the medical treatment'.[20] Bible readings and prayers were held morning and evening on the wards and Theodor Fliedner advised the deaconesses on how to draw their patients into religious discussion.[21] In an 1873 letter to a young woman interested in training as a nurse, Nightingale wrote:

> I could not recommend Kaiserswerth, even if they would receive you. The spirit of the place is beautiful – But as a Hospital it is so inferior to any London Hospital, where you see more real work in a week than you do at Kaiserswerth in a year.[22]

---

2011).

[17]  Nightingale, *The Institution*, p. 27; WI/Ms/9025/67–8.

[18]  DK/FA/X1; Sticker, *Theodor Fliedner and Nursing*, p. 7; see, for example, E. White, 'The German Hospital – a Unique Story', *History of Nursing Journal*, 3/2 (1990): pp. 24–5.

[19]  Baly, *Florence Nightingale*, p. 219.

[20]  LMA H01/ST/NC1/66/24.6.

[21]  Nightingale, *The Institution*, p. 17.

[22]  LMA/H01/ST/NC3/SU211.

This was the crux of Nightingale's many criticisms of Kaiserswerth – it was a medical backwater. The primary focus was on its religious mission.

The deaconesses' nursing training was a minor part of their overall programme; they also had to do a significant amount of cleaning, but nevertheless it was training, and it was systematic. Most training occurred on the hospital wards, although they also undertook nursing in the local community. By 1850 the probationers had a one-hour nursing class a week, seven hours of Bible studies, plus lessons in reading, writing, arithmetic, needlework and singing. Sister Gertrude Reichardt, the first Kaiserswerth deaconess and the only one not to serve a probation period, taught the nursing class. When she entered Kaiserswerth, she was already an experienced nurse, having assisted her father and brother, who were both physicians. The deaconesses learnt nine nursing competencies: dressing wounds; smearing and laying on mustard and other plasters; bathing, rubbing and using a thermometer (most likely to test the bath water); giving enemas; applying leeches; cupping; laying out the dead, and a knowledge of herbs.[23] They were also trained as apothecaries in the Kaiserswerth dispensary, and were examined and licensed as dispensers by the government medical officer.

On the whole, learning nursing at Kaiserswerth was a true apprentice experience. Probationers observed procedures being carried out by an experienced nurse, and then were supervised doing them before performing them on their own. Most of the time the probationers worked with an experienced nurse, but they were also occasionally in charge. Even as short-term foreign visitors, Florence Nightingale was in charge one day and Agnes Jones some evenings. Nurses took turns on the night watch. As befitted a religious institution, supervision was strict. The sister in charge of the probationers kept a weekly record of each probationer. This record noted each probationer's hospital ward assignment, learning, character and conduct. She was judged on cleanliness, order, industry, sincerity, peaceableness, obedience and serious conduct.[24] Serious or sober conduct, as the Victorians more often put it, meant not only non-drunken, but quiet, modest, purposeful behaviour.

There were many obvious ways in which the Kaiserswerth system, which shared many features with the Catholic nursing sisterhoods, was copied by nurse training schools in London and worldwide. The programmes began with a probationary period, and consisted mostly of ward work, supplemented by a little formal classroom teaching. Students were rotated through various wards. There were lists of skills to be learnt and character traits that were judged. Later nurses' homes all had residences under the control of a house mother or 'home sister'. But it was one thing to establish this system in a small religious institution under the guiding vision of its founders, and quite another to insert that system into large traditional unsectarian teaching hospitals under the control of all-male boards and doctors.

---

[23] WI/Mss/9025/68, 71 and 84.
[24] WI/Ms/9084/7.

A major stumbling block to the whole nursing reform enterprise in London related to the recruitment of suitable persons. Nightingale acknowledged on her first visit to Kaiserswerth that Theodor Fliedner had recruited the right kind of women and influenced them in the right way so that he could trust them with the spiritual care of the hospital patients.[25] But he was recruiting women with religious motivation, and he was recruiting at a time of demographic and social upheaval in Germany when young single women were looking for work.[26] These characteristics of the Kaiserswerth venture could not easily be transported to other countries, such as England, and to unsectarian contexts. Yet the Kaiserswerth model was hugely attractive to an English audience largely because it presented a *Protestant*, *genteel* experience. Hospital boards were quick to see the advantage of its major characteristic: a cheap, conscientious labour pool. As we will see in later chapters, they soon turned the system to their advantage.

### The Institution of Nursing Sisters: The Importance of Hospital Training and Better Living Conditions

In May 1840 the Quaker philanthropist Elizabeth Fry visited the Kaiserswerth Diakoniewerk for one or two days. This brief visit inspired her to found the Protestant Sisters of Charity, the first English Protestant organization to offer nurses some rudimentary training. Fry wished to develop an 'altogether different and superior' class of nurses, by which she meant a more respectable group of working-class nurses rather than women from a higher social class.[27] Because it was unacceptable for Victorian ladies to transact business with men in the public sphere, the new organization had a Ladies' Committee which managed the household, while a Gentlemen's Committee dealt with business matters. Although Fry's nurses were called 'sisters', they were not sisters in either the sense of being members of a religious sisterhood or in the nursing sense of head nurses. Because many people mistakenly identified them with the Catholic order of the Sisters of Charity, in 1842 the Ladies' Committee changed the name from the Protestant Sisters of Charity to the Institution of Nursing Sisters. The Fry nurses were also frequently called Mrs Fry's Sisters, and after they moved to Devonshire Square in 1842, the Devonshire Square Sisters.

Members of the institution signed a contract agreeing to work for three years. They then spent a probationary period from several weeks to three months working in teaching hospitals such as the London, Guy's and St George's, and later, St Thomas'. They received no formal instruction, but picked up what they could from

---

25    Nightingale, *The Institution*, p. 7.

26    C.M. Prelinger, *Charity, Challenge, and Change: Religious Dimensions of the Mid-nineteenth-century Women's Movement in Germany* (New York, 1987), p. 21.

27    K. Fry and R.E. Cresswell (eds), *Memoirs of the Life of Elizabeth Fry* (2 vols, Philadelphia, PA, 1848), vol. 2, p. 405.

the hospital nurses. In 1844 the Ladies' Committee sent the matron at St George's a list of duties in which they wanted the probationers instructed, but whether the hospital sisters followed through is not recorded.[28]

Reforming hospital nursing was not Fry's aim. Rather, her nurses worked primarily for private patients, who paid the organization, and for poor patients, gratis. Occasionally, the nurses worked as head nurses in hospitals such as Guy's, the London and the German Hospital.[29] The Society paid the sisters £20 a year, rising to £23 after three years, with full board and uniform provided. The patients paid the institution, not the individual nurse, £1 a week for an experienced nurse. Although hospitals paid only about half the rate private patients paid – for example, in 1842 the London Hospital paid the institution £22 a year for a head nurse, as opposed to £52 private patients would have paid – the Ladies' Committee recognized that hospital experience was advantageous, and therefore accepted the lower wage in a few selected cases.[30]

Fry and her Ladies' Committee[31] appreciated that good living and working conditions were essential if they wished to attract respectable women; visitors must not be able to wander in and out of the nurses' dormitories at will as they did at Guy's. The probationers did not usually live in the miserable hospital quarters when they were in training, but rather in the comfortable nurses' home where the sisters also lived when they were not out on their cases. In 1842 the institution stopped sending their nurses to the London Hospital for training because they thought it was too dirty.[32] In 1843, Lady Inglis, a Ladies' Committee member and later chair, advised that the duties – presumably the cleaning – and the low pay at the Middlesex Hospital disqualified it as an employer for Fry nurses.[33] The Institution of Nursing Sisters gave its nurses two weeks annual leave in 1850 and established a pension fund to which the ladies contributed £1,000 in 1853.[34]

The women who entered the Institution of Nursing Sisters as probationers were typical of the old nurses: they were primarily older women in dire circumstances. Mary Taylor was a 37-year-old widow with two children, one dependent on her. Jane Francis was a 46-year-old widow with two children, one in service and one

---

[28]   WI/SA/QNI/W2/2, 23 February, 22 March, 3 May 1844, 18 July 1845.

[29]   The German Hospital was founded in 1845, primarily for German immigrants in London, and was nursed by Kaiserswerth deaconesses.

[30]   R.G. Huntsman, M. Bruin and D. Holttum, 'Twixt Candle and Lamp: The Contribution of Elizabeth Fry and the Institution of Nursing Sisters to Nursing Reform', *Medical History*, 46/3 (2002): pp. 360–61, 374; WI/SA/QNI/W2/3, 29 January 1846, 21 August 1847.

[31]   Although Elizabeth Fry remained nominally president until her death in 1845, her sister-in-law, Mrs Elizabeth Gurney, did the major part of running the institution. Fry and Cresswell, *Memoirs of the Life of Elizabeth Fry*, vol. 2, p. 405.

[32]   WI/SA/QNI/W2/1, 16 and 29 July, 28 August 1842.

[33]   WI/SA/QNI/W2/2, 18 August 1843.

[34]   WI/SA/QNI/W2/3, 1 February 1850; WI/SA/QNI/W2/4, 9 December 1853.

dependent on her. The widowed Mary Godfrey was 50 years old and had four children, two of whom were dependent on her. Sarah Holland was a 38-year-old widow who claimed to have been in 'circumstances of much comfort' before the death of her husband. She was cheerful, efficient, attentive and obliging, but was dismissed in December 1842 for coming home drunk.[35]

The organization grew gradually: in 1844 there were only 14 nurses, in 1847 there were 26, and in 1861, 71 nurses.[36] As more women applied, the ladies were able to be more selective.[37] By 1846 a number of experienced hospital nurses began joining the institution. Ann Jones, Mary Saunders and Anne Fisher came from Guy's.[38] Mrs Taylor, who had been a nurse at the Westminster and King's College Hospitals, was accepted in May 1847.[39] She may very possibly have been Mary Anne Taylor, the clinically competent nurse whom, in January 1846, the Westminster had fired for her terrible temper and tyrannical behaviour. Most of the sisters were successful. Jane Francis, one of the first nurses to join the organization, was kind and attentive and, one surgeon reported, managed a degree of cleanliness in a case of nervous debility which he thought remarkable under the circumstances. Eliza Dowman's 'knowledge and experience (which are great)', one referee wrote, 'are more than equalled by her judicious and humane attentions'.[40]

Despite the ladies' careful screening, they did have to discharge a number of nurses for all the standard problems: leaving their patients untended for long blocks of time, staying out all night, unkindness to the patients, impropriety, and most often, drunkenness.[41] Like many accomplished nurses, Eliza Dowman was fond of drink, and was later fired for staying out all night and enticing other sisters to visit public houses.[42] Other problems arose because members of the aristocracy used Fry's nurses, and occasionally there were complaints that the nurses were used to nursing 'very high and wealthy families' and were 'uncomfortable and unpleasant with persons in less affluent circumstances'.[43] Dr Henry Bence Jones of St George's Hospital made a rare complaint when he said Jane Medwinter was far from being a first-rate nurse because she had insufficient physical strength and judgement, although he admitted, grudgingly, that she followed his orders.

[35] WI/SA/QNI/W4, pp. 2–4, 13; WI/SA/QNI/W5, p. 16; WI/SA/QNI/W2/2, 2 December 1842.

[36] WI/SA/QNI/W2/2, 12 July 1844; Huntsman et al., 'Twixt Candle and Lamp', p. 360; LMA/H01/ST/NC16/5, p. 11.

[37] See, for example, WI/SA/QNI/W2/3, 24 September 1847.

[38] WI/SA/QNI/W2/3, 17 April, 15 and 29 May 1846.

[39] WI/SA/QNI/W2/3, 23 April and 7 May 1847.

[40] WI/SA/QNI/W5, pp. 2, 63.

[41] WI/SA/QNI/W2/1, 18 February, 17 June, 18 November, 2 December 1842, 22 September 1843, 12 and 26 January, 3 May 1844; see also Huntsman et al., 'Twixt Candle and Lamp', p. 371.

[42] WI/SA/QNI/W2/2, 7 May, 9 August, 13 December 1844.

[43] WI/SA/QNI/W5, pp. 7, 61; WI/SA/QNI/W2/2, 7 February, 7 March 1845.

Medwinter was reproved for refusing to attend a poor patient, and then, although she had very good references mentioning her propriety, energy and kindness, dismissed in 1846 for unkindness, leaving a patient after an operation and staying out all night.[44]

When Nightingale went to Scutari in October 1854 during the Crimean War, she tried to recruit Fry nurses. The Ladies' Committee at first refused to let any go, but in 1855 they sent three. The first was Amelia Lamacroft, who gave general satisfaction and conducted herself with strict propriety. The second, Lucy Church, was an excellent nurse with thoroughly good principles and very respectful to her superiors. The third, Anne Harnack, was considered respectable but inefficient. Later in the war, another three Fry sisters were sent to the naval hospital at Therapia, where they did well.[45]

The smattering of hospital training and the improved living conditions and benefits Fry's Sisters received enabled her institution to recruit and retain some skilled, respectable nurses. However, it had been designed largely as a private nursing agency. The matron who lived with the nurses in the home was not a nurse, and there was no centralized training school as at Kaiserswerth and in the Catholic convents. Rather, the probationers received a decentralized, hit-and-miss training from a variety of sisters in different hospitals. Nor could the Institution for Nursing Sisters produce the large supply of trained nurses which the new hospital medicine required; the largest number ever on the institution's roster was only about 100.[46] Still, Elizabeth Fry's nurses had shown that, given better conditions, it was possible to produce respectable, skilled nurses, albeit largely domiciliary nurses.

**The Hospital for Gentlewomen: The Failure of a German Model**

When, in the winter of 1853, the Ladies' Committee of the Establishment for Gentlewomen during Temporary Illness asked Florence Nightingale if she would consider being their lady superintendent, she was keenly interested. Nightingale had returned from Kaiserswerth in 1850 deeply impressed by the 'delicacy, the cheerfulness, the grace of Christian kindness, the moral atmosphere' which pervaded its hospital. By contrast, she thought the English hospitals 'almost a school for impropriety and immorality'. At Kaiserswerth there were five male nurses in the men's wards so that no sister was asked to do anything but what a lady in a private house would do for her brother. Physical examinations of female patients were conducted in privacy. The Sisters read family prayers in their wards

---

[44]    WI/SA/QNI/W5, pp. 55, 80, 99; WI/SA/QNI/W2/2, 7 February 1845; WI/SA/QNI/W2/3, 17 April 1846.

[45]    WI/SA/QNI/W2/4, 20 October 1854; LMA/H01/ST/NC8/1, pp. 17–18; WI/SA/QNI/W2/4, 9 February 1855, 25 April, 29 August 1856.

[46]    Huntsman et al., 'Twixt Candle and Lamp', pp. 362–3.

each morning and evening, generally sang a hymn with the patients, and then read them a short portion of the Bible.[47] In the men's wards in the London hospitals the nurses were all women. The sisters were supposed to read morning and evening prayers, but did not always do so. Physical examinations of women and all but life-threatening operations were conducted on the wards, in full view of the other patients.[48] Nightingale thought the Gentlewomen's Hospital would be a good place to establish a Kaiserswerth type of training school for nurses. The year she spent at this small hospital demonstrates the underlying difficulties in transferring a German model to a London hospital in the 1850s.

Lady Charlotte Canning and a group of philanthropic ladies had founded the Gentlewomen's Hospital in 1849 at 8 Chandos Street, Cavendish Square. Like Fry's institution, it had a Ladies' and a Gentlemen's Committee. Its patients were 'educated women', as Nightingale described them, largely governesses, 'too poor to obtain medical assistance or come to London for that purpose, too refined to go into the [public] hospitals',[49] but most were able to contribute something towards their care.

The hospital had not prospered. The ladies could not find efficient nurses, and had to rely on temporary nurses from Fry's institution and St John's House.[50] In June 1850 the ladies questioned whether they really needed two nurses and an under-nurse for six patients, and commented that the nurses needed 'to be spoken to'.[51] The Ladies' Committee gave Mrs Willingate, a Fry nurse, a good character when she left, but later discovered that she had been drunk on several occasions, was frequently negligent and unkind to the patients, and habitually stayed out without leave very late in the evening.[52] In July 1852 the ladies asked the matron to keep a closer eye on the servants[53] – another indication of the difficulties of a committee trying to run even a very small hospital without a competent matron.

This lack of a competent matron was a key problem. Although the wealthy and influential Ladies' Committee paid their matrons extremely well, they were unable to find an able one. In 1850 the matron's salary was £50 a year with board and laundry.[54] By contrast, in 1854, University College, King's College and St Mary's Hospitals paid their new matrons the same amount, but the ladies' hospital had a maximum of six patients, while the matrons of the other hospitals were

---

[47]   Nightingale, *The Institution*, pp. 15, 19–20, citation on p. 15.

[48]   See, for example, LMA/H09/GY/A67/4/1, 15 January 1868.

[49]   BL 45796, fol. 134.

[50]   See, for example, FNM/HSP/Agenda Book, 13 May, 3 and 10 June 1850, 6 January 1851, 16 February 1852, 11 February 1853. We are indebted to Professor Louise Selanders for informing us of this new acquisition of the Florence Nightingale Museum.

[51]   FNM/HSP/Agenda Book, 17 June, 15 July 1850.

[52]   FNM/HSP/Letter Book, 28 July [1851].

[53]   FNM/HSP/Agenda Book, 23 July 1852.

[54]   Ibid., 7 June [1850].

responsible for approximately 80–100.[55] The first matron, Miss Hall, was an experienced matron who was kind and attentive to the patients, but only days after she started in March 1850, the ladies dismissed her. The ladies thought: 'A longer period of trial would in all probability lead to disappointment and difficulty.'[56] They began considering discharging the second matron, Miss Woolley, in July 1851, and finally gave her notice in October.[57] When Woolley left at the end of December 1851, the ladies redefined the position and searched for a 'lady superintendent' who would be competent to handle the 'details of management', allowing the Ladies' Committee to deal with the accounts and act as an admissions committee. They changed the duties of the cook and housekeeper to accommodate this arrangement, and asked Miss Helps to be the lady superintendent.

Helps was one of the three original St John's House Sisters, and had been acting lady superintendent there at various times. She had left the sisterhood in September 1851, and in 1852 was travelling on the Continent with her sister. She declined the appointment.[58] Helps is an illustration of how small and close-knit the nursing reform community was. Lady Inglis, chair of the Ladies' Committee of Fry's institution, was also a member of the Ladies' Committee of the Hospital for Gentlewomen.[59] The Bishop of London, Charles James Blomfield, one of the two principal founders of St John's House, was a patron who, from the founding of the Gentlewomen's Hospital, gave it his 'fostering care and judicious advice'.[60] The hospital seems to have run with no matron, then a temporary matron from the end of May 1852,[61] when Miss Wilkinson was appointed.[62] One of the ladies later described Wilkinson as a disreputable character.[63]

Nightingale made a striking contrast to the previous matrons. Most unusually, she had both the status of a lady and clinical nursing experience. She had read hospital reports extensively, visited numerous hospitals in Britain and on the Continent,[64] and of course, trained at Kaiserswerth. The Ladies' Committee hoped that with so able a superintendent, the hospital would become more successful. In 1850, Nightingale had visited Berlin, where the greater social freedom which young ladies like her deaconess friend Marianne von Rantzau enjoyed made a deep

[55]   LMA/H02/WH/A1/37, 27 February 1855.

[56]   FNM/HSP/Letter Book, 25 March [1850].

[57]   Ibid., 24 October 1851; FNM/HSP/Agenda Book, 7, 17 and 28 July 1851.

[58]   LMA/H01/ST/SJ/A19/1, 2 June 1849; LMA/H01/ST/SJ/A19/2, 21 July 1849, 6 April 1850, 29 September 1851; FNM/HSP/Agenda Book, 3 and 7 November, 5 December 1851.

[59]   FNM/HSP/Letter Book, 22 April 1853.

[60]   FNM/HSP/Agenda Book, 15 March 1852; FNM/HSP, *The Pen*, 1/7 (1853): 'Benevolent Institutions', p. 103.

[61]   Ibid., 16, 19 and 26 April, 14 and 21 May 1852.

[62]   Ibid., 31 May 1852.

[63]   BL 45790, fol. 148.

[64]   Cook, *The Life of Florence Nightingale*, vol. 1, pp. 127–8.

impression on her. Young unmarried ladies could walk about unchaperoned and even answer their front door themselves. Furthermore, they could maintain their status as ladies while working full-time, albeit unpaid, as nursing superintendents. Von Rantzau had trained for a year at Kaiserswerth and then founded and ran the Bethanien Hospital on the Kaiserswerth plan. The deaconesses came from all social classes – the nobility, the middle class and farm girls. Nightingale judged it a model hospital.

'The hospital is like a palace – the deaconesses' rooms are just like ours at Embley[65] and the superintendent has her two rooms with books and prints and flowers,' Nightingale enthused, 'just as I think the intellectual and practical life ought to be always combined.' Von Rantzau took Nightingale to two other Berlin hospitals which ladies superintended, one of which von Rantzau thought better than the Bethanien. 'There is no more question about immorality there than there is in private families in England,' Nightingale reassured her parents, 'and the licentiousness of the medical class is just as much put a stop to as it is in our homes. In fact, the great difficulties of hospitals disappear altogether.' In Nightingale's view, the Prussians thought hospitals should be 'schools of moral influence for the patients'.[66]

It was once thought that Nightingale had no definite plans for nursing reform until the Crimean War,[67] but when she replied to the Ladies' Committee in February 1853, she outlined in detail how, if she did accept the position, she would reorganize the hospital and use it as a training school for nurses. 'The future object, of course,' she told the ladies, 'will be to train sisters to undertake wards in the London public hospitals.'[68] After Nightingale agreed to be lady superintendent, the speakers at the hospital's public meeting in July 1853 emphasized that the hospital was to be a training centre for efficient nurses, both paid and volunteer. Sir James Kay-Shuttleworth explained that the board hoped to:

> send forth a totally different class of nurses from those who were to be found in public hospitals. It would be exceedingly revolting to the feelings of a Christian public if they were made generally aware of the state of things which existed in some of the hospitals. The superior nurses in these establishments were often women of good character, and considerable skill, but the assistants were generally low, disorderly, and almost sottish women ....

Some hospitals, Kay-Shuttleworth continued, engaged nurses without checking references, so that, after being fired by one hospital, these women simply moved to another.[69] Kay-Shuttleworth is best known for his work as a civil servant reforming

---

[65]    Embley was the grander of the two Nightingale country homes.

[66]    Claydon House Archives, Bundle 122, Nightingale to her family, July 1850.

[67]    Dingwall et al., *An Introduction to the Social History of Nursing*, p. 49.

[68]    LMA/H01/ST/NC5/3/3, fol. 11.

[69]    FNM/HSP, 'Benevolent Institutions', pp. 100, 102, citation on p. 102.

education, but he spoke from first-hand experience, for he had qualified as a doctor at Edinburgh and practised medicine for eight years before moving into the civil service.[70] Dr Henry Bence Jones, a consultant at the Hospital for Gentlewomen, responded that low, disorderly nurses were not knowingly suffered at his hospital, St George's. There was certainly 'abundant room for improvement', but board members visited the patients periodically and questioned them to see if they had any complaints. Any serious charge was instantly followed by suspension and, when the next Weekly Committee met, dismissal.[71] Kay-Shuttleworth attested to the progress the ward system had made by mid-century in creating some skilled and respectable sisters, while both he and Bence Jones indicated the lack of headway made with the assistant nurses.

If she accepted the position, Nightingale planned to assume the right to discharge nurses without consulting the board. In a plan she never implemented, she gave considerable thought to improving the nurses' characters. She discussed how she would install a 'Mother' similar to Caroline Fliedner to have the moral guardianship of the whole concern. There would be volunteer unpaid sisters from all classes, and a chaplain to give the sisters Bible instruction three evenings a week. Every sister was to sing, pray and read the scriptures in her ward twice a day. The chaplain would direct the sisters' choice of readings: 'Should the chaplain be such a man as can direct her, she may besides keep in a book a weekly account of each patient's conduct and dispositions, to be shown to the chaplain only or to the Mother.' Because Nightingale expected that, as at Kaiserswerth, many probationers would be uneducated, a sister would give the under-nurses 'lessons in reading, writing, arithmetic, needlework, geography, and also scriptural instruction from 10–12 am and from 8–9 pm every day'. Nightingale added: 'It would greatly tend to making the devotions in each ward agreeable to the patients, if the nurses were also instructed in singing.' The House Surgeon would give instructions in 'small matters such as dressing wounds', but, Nightingale insisted, 'the surgeon must never be master of the institution'.[72]

Thus far, Nightingale followed the Kaiserswerth model closely, but she also made some major changes. At Kaiserswerth the Sisters did all the cleaning, while Nightingale planned on hiring a maid to cook and clean the house. The most striking change was Nightingale's appropriation of the dominant role Fliedner played at Kaiserswerth.[73] She had insisted that she would choose the new house for the hospital, appoint the chaplain, and manage the hospital's funds. 'Unless I am left a free agent and am to organise the thing myself and not they [the Ladies' Committee],' she concluded, 'I will have nothing to do with it.'[74] Important as the

---

[70]  R.J.W. Selleck, *James Kay-Shuttleworth: Journey of an Outsider* (Ilford, Essex, 1994), pp. 42–5, 100–101.

[71]  FNM/HSP, 'Benevolent Institutions', p. 103.

[72]  WI/Mss/8994/89; LMA/H01/ST/NC5/3/3.

[73]  Nightingale, *The Institution*, pp. 16–17, 20.

[74]  BL 43397, fol. 306.

role of the Harley Street chaplain was to be for the religious training of the staff, he was definitely not to be in charge. Nightingale accordingly selected 'good, harmless Mr. Garnier' as chaplain.[75]

Nightingale formally accepted the position of unpaid lady superintendent on 28 April 1853.[76] She immediately consulted Miss Elizabeth Frere, the first lady superintendent of St John's House.[77] Frere suggested changes in the hospital rules which further increased the authority of the lady superintendent. Nightingale adopted her suggestions wholesale, and also wrote into the contract that she could retire within a year if she found the hospital unsuitable as a training school for nurses.[78]

In June 1853 the ladies agreed to occupy a new larger house, able to accommodate 27 patients, at 1 Upper Harley Street.[79] Before Nightingale took up residence on 12 August 1853,[80] she was receiving 'a quantity of offers of Sisters', most of whom she considered completely unsuitable. One was a cousin of a German acquaintance who appeared in London without warning and informed Nightingale she was going to join her at Harley Street. When Nightingale finally convinced her that this was not possible, the lady quietly told her she would stay in London for a year to see. She was a very handsome woman with the sweetest voice she had ever heard, Nightingale wrote, but spoke no English.[81]

In September Nightingale had three probationary sisters,[82] but the only probationary sister referred to by name is her cousin Bertha Smith who arrived later, in November, 'to assist her as a "Nursing Sister"'.[83] As there is no further mention of her at Harley Street, it is unlikely she stayed for long. When Smith later offered to join Nightingale at Scutari, Nightingale replied: 'We think it quite out of the question to have dear Bertha here. It is not a place for her indeed.'[84] Nevertheless, Nightingale originally had great hopes for the volunteer sister system: 'How happy I will be when we have all sisters!', she wrote to Pastor Fliedner.[85] But after September, with the one exception of Bertha Smith, there is no mention of any probationary sisters in the surviving records.

Nightingale had the same difficulties with the paid nurses as the earlier matrons. They gave her 'infinite trouble' because, she complained, they had 'neither love

---

75    WI/Ms/8994/80; BL 45790, fol. 155.

76    FNM/HSP/Agenda Book, 28 April 1852.

77    Columbia University School of Nursing Nightingale Collection, C-5.

78    BL 45796, fol. 22.

79    BL 45796, fol. 39; Sir H. Verney (ed.), *Florence Nightingale at Harley Street: Her Reports to the Governors of Her Nursing Home 1853–4* (London, 1970), p. 6.

80    Ibid., p viii.

81    WI/Ms/8994/32.

82    DK/FA/I/K/b3 (in French).

83    FNM//HSP/Agenda Book, 18 November 1853; WI/Ms/8994/57.

84    WI/Ms/8995/23.

85    DK/FA/II/K/b3.

nor conscience'.[86] She feared that a Fry nurse was not working out, and she gave warning to another nurse because she knew nothing about nursing.[87] In October, when a major operation was under way on the ground floor, the patients on the first floor 'rebelled' against their nurse, forcing Nightingale to replace her.[88] The following May, Nightingale dismissed another nurse because of 'her love of opium and intimidation'.[89]

With the exception of one nurse, Theresa Foster,[90] whom Nightingale had paid St John's House to train and who, as a result, refused to do any work other than nursing,[91] Nightingale used the paid nurses in the traditional way as maids-of-all-work. In her first three months she hired no charwoman, needlewoman or night nurse, but used the day nurses to do this work. Nurse Smith helped to piece together used carpets from the Chandos Street building, and Nurse Harding did laundry and helped make the outfit for one of the scrofulous[92] patients who was emigrating to New Zealand.[93] Nevertheless, the nurses had reasonable living and working conditions and good pay, originally £16 16s. a year, which Nightingale increased to £20 and £25,[94] presumably with all found.[95] Under her direction, two to three nurses looked after 9–17 patients. In comparison, a King's College Hospital nurse, who made £12 in her first year and £14 from then on, looked after up to 15 patients.[96] At St George's in 1853, assistant nurses started at £16 and head nurses at £20 a year, with no increase for three years.[97]

Although the hospital was designed for gentlewomen with *temporary* illnesses, Nightingale soon realized that many of the patients had chronic diseases.[98] As in most hospitals, two months was the allowed length of stay, but the patients continually asked, and were allowed, to stay longer.[99] Sick women with low incomes were unlikely to have alternative homes which befitted their self-concept

[86]    Ibid.

[87]    Leeds District Archives, Wyas, Canning/177/2/5, 13 September 1853. She had also fired the under-housemaid.

[88]    WI/Ms/8994/49.

[89]    Verney, *Florence Nightingale at Harley Street*, p. 28.

[90]    LMA/H01/ST/SJ/A20/2, 18 July, 26 September 1853. Foster was sometimes spelled 'Forster'.

[91]    WI/Ms/8994/57.

[92]    Scrofula, often called the King's Evil, was a disease producing swollen glands, often caused by tuberculosis.

[93]    Verney, *Florence Nightingale at Harley Street*, p. 3.

[94]    FNM//HSP/Agenda Book, 2 May, 7 November 1853.

[95]    'All found' meant that in addition to the monetary payment, the employer paid the employee's room, board, uniforms and washing.

[96]    KH/CM/M3, 20 December 1850; KH/CM/M2, 5 April 1843.

[97]    SGH/MBG, 16 February, 23 March 1853.

[98]    WI/Ms/8994/47.

[99]    FNM//HSP/Agenda Book, passim.

as gentlewomen, and by December Nightingale was convinced that many of her patients tried to prolong their hospital stay as long as possible. Nightingale thought they made the most of their respite: 'Gentility & eating & drinking (more particularly drinking, wine or spirits)', she wrote, were their main concerns.[100] To her father, she complained that 'This place is exactly like the administering of the Poor Law.' Some patients had 'purely lazy fits', while others had been abandoned by their families.[101] Nightingale subscribed to the philosophy enshrined in the 1834 Poor Law: providing too much assistance encouraged people to become permanently dependent on welfare.[102] If the hospital was too attractive, she feared that most of her patients would make illness an amusement and a luxury for want of any higher interest in life, or their families would use the hospital as the cheapest way of supporting them.[103] Such patients also did not give her nurses adequate clinical experience. She convinced the Ladies' Committee to limit admissions to cases of serious illness.[104] The impact of this policy was soon felt. While she had 17 patients in February 1854,[105] from March 15 to May 15 the hospital averaged only nine patients.[106]

Nightingale's contract specified she could leave after one year if she found the hospital unsuitable for a training school, and from the beginning she had planned to stay at Harley Street only a few years. She then hoped to 'try the real work in a better soil, that of a public infirmary'.[107] This opportunity presented itself in July 1854, when King's College Hospital approached her to take over its nursing service. In her quarterly report on 7 August 1854, Nightingale informed the Ladies' Committee:

> I have not effected anything towards the object of training nurses – my primary idea in devoting my life to Hospital work for, owing to the small number of applications, the Committee have not been able to select, in all cases, proper objects for Medical & Surgical treatment – and accordingly the result has not been satisfactory to me.

If she could find a situation which would enable her to start a nursing school, she would leave, giving three to six months' notice.[108] Nightingale could not explain

---

[100]  Verney, *Florence Nightingale at Harley Street*, pp. 16–17 (emphases in original).

[101]  BL Add Mss 45790 f 156; WI/Ms/8994/80.

[102]  R.K. Webb, *Modern England from The Eighteenth Century to the Present* (2nd edn, London, 1980), pp. 247–8.

[103]  WI/Ms/8994/84.

[104]  Verney, *Florence Nightingale at Harley Street*, p. 18.

[105]  WI/Ms/8994/96.

[106]  Verney, *Florence Nightingale at Harley Street*, p. 27; BL 43402, fol. 154.

[107]  DK/FA/II/K/b3.

[108]  Verney, *Florence Nightingale at Harley Street*, pp. 35–6, citation on p. 35; See also WI/Ms/8994/111.

that she was then in negotiations with King's College Hospital for precisely such a position because the hospital's committee had asked her to keep the negotiations secret.[109] These negotiations were aborted in October when the War Department asked her to take a party of government-paid nurses to Scutari.

At Harley Street, Nightingale had none of the problems which hobbled the old matrons. She was extraordinarily competent, well-versed in nursing, and had full control of her staff and the hospital itself. She had the complete confidence of the attending doctors and the Ladies' and Gentlemen's Committees, and under her direction the hospital was eminently respectable. Although she ran the institution at a substantial deficit, this does not seem to have been a major problem with her wealthy and influential board.

Nightingale gave the cause for her inability to establish a training school as the lack of a critical mass of patients and the paucity of acute care patients. In short, like Kaiserswerth, she considered Harley Street a medical backwater. She did not mention the second major hurdle she had been unable to surmount: the difficulty of attracting suitable probationers, and especially unpaid probationary sisters. Despite major modifications to the Kaiserswerth model, it was not suited to the English social structure. Victorian conventions placed greater constraints on young ladies; they did not have the freedom of action of their German counterparts whose independence had so impressed Nightingale. Competent English ladies drew back from performing what they considered the menial, drudging work of nursing, 'sweeping, combing out dirty heads' and 'dressing loathsome wounds', as Nightingale described it.[110] Furthermore, working side-by-side with working-class nurses was simply not appropriate for ladies in the class-bound society of England in the 1850s. When, in the summer of 1854, Nightingale began devising plans for training nurses at King's College Hospital, she had given up trying to attract women from the upper classes, and instead planned to recruit such sturdy working-class women as farmers' daughters.[111] A third barrier to her planned training school, and perhaps the most important, was the reputation English hospitals and their nurses had earned for impropriety and immorality. The real difficulty, Nightingale wrote in 1861, this time referring to the Nightingale Training School, was to find respectable persons willing to be sisters.[112]

## Conclusion

While Elizabeth Fry's nursing institution made real headway in developing respectable nurses, the Fry nurses were primarily domiciliary nurses. Nightingale had been unable to establish a training school at the Harley Street hospital, and

---

[109]   WI/Mss/8994/107 and 110.
[110]   Nightingale, *The Institution*, pp. 18–19.
[111]   Cook, *The Life of Florence Nightingale*, vol. 1, p. 141.
[112]   DK/II/K/b3.

neither institution was able to produce the large numbers of skilled nurses the teaching hospitals required. Kaiserswerth did train large numbers of competent nurses whom it sent all over the world, but it was a German institution, and the model did not take root in English soil. A primary obstacle was securing adequate funding – a problem which would continue to be a major issue throughout the history of nursing – but the biggest hurdle in the 1850s was the social reputation of the teaching hospitals and their nurses. At mid-century, most people still considered nursing a disreputable occupation. Yet real improvements had been made, as the Crimean War in 1854–56 would reveal. That war provides a case study of the different types and abilities of British nurses at mid-century.

# Chapter 5

# Nursing at the Crossroads, Part 1: Ladies and Religious Sisters in the Crimean War

The British women who nursed in the military hospitals during the Crimean War from 1854 to 1856 provide a prosopographical illustration of the state of nursing reform and nursing practice in the 1850s. The British government had declared war on Russia in March 1854, and in October, in response to a fierce public outcry over the lack of care for wounded and dying soldiers, sent 38 government-paid nurses under the direction of Florence Nightingale to the army's two base hospitals in Scutari, Turkey. Eight further parties of nurses followed, and nine more base hospitals opened in both Turkey and Russia.[1]

The records of five different lady superintendents have survived: Nightingale, who was lady superintendent of the two Scutari hospitals, and for some months of the Balaclava General Hospital; Mary Stanley and Emily Hutton at the Koulali Hospitals; Henrietta LeMesurier at the Smyrna Hospital, and Maria Parkes at the Renkioi Hospital. In addition, Selena Bracebridge, Nightingale's friend and chaperone in Scutari, often made comments in the ladies' records. The records of other lady superintendents – for example, Mrs Holmes Coutt at the Smyrna Hospital, or Mother Emma Langston, Margaret Wear and Sister Bertha Turnbull, all superintendents for short periods at the Balaclava General Hospital – have not survived.

While the information these ladies give us is the best we have about nursing practice at mid-century, it has major gaps and serious biases. First, some of the 11 hospitals in which the government nurses worked in Turkey and the Crimea were hundreds of miles apart;[2] some were not under Nightingale's direction; the lady superintendents changed from time to time, and as new hospitals opened and others closed, nurses were moved from one to another. Second, the working-class nurses were not representative of their class; they were considered the very best nurses because they were carefully chosen from a huge number of applicants. All the hospital nurses came with good references from matrons, doctors and/

---

[1]   W. Baumgart, *The Crimean War 1853–56* (London, 1999), pp. 14, 143–4; FNM/ LMA/H1/ST/NC8/1.

[2]   Five hospitals were in Turkey: two in Scutari (the Barrack and the General Hospitals), two in Koulali (the Upper and the Lower Hospitals), and the Palace Hospital for officers in Kadekoi. In the Crimea, there were four: the Balaclava General, the Castle, the Land Transport and the Monastery Hospitals. In addition, there were two civil or civilian hospitals in Turkey, one in Renkioi and the second in Smyrna.

or chaplains.[3] Third, only one working-class nurse, Elizabeth Davis, wrote her own story.[4] Her autobiography, written with the help of a professional journalist and supported by women who were hostile to Nightingale and had launched a frivolous libel suit against her, is a somewhat suspect source. Davis nevertheless gives us a real sense of the spirit and values of an experienced working-class nurse. Otherwise, we must rely on the perspectives of three ladies who published memoirs of their war experiences, the five lady superintendents and Bracebridge mentioned above who wrote references for the nurses after the end of the war, and the diaries of four Catholic Sisters of Mercy. Feeling it would be disrespectful, these ladies frequently did not write references for women of their own class, and they sometimes did not comment on dismissed nurses.

The six ladies looked at the nurses from a standard upper-class perspective and sometimes had different personal opinions of them. For example, Maria Parkes and Henrietta LeMesurier both judged Miss Warens, who worked in Renkioi and Smyrna, a good nurse, but Parkes considered her a foolish woman, while LeMesurier thought her clever.[5] Selena Bracebridge was by far the harshest, and also the least reliable, of the nurses' evaluators. Like many upper-class women of her day, she looked down on the nurses, expecting complete submissiveness and deference from them. She was also afraid of what her class considered the violent tendencies of the working classes. She thought Mrs McPhee 'very impudent in conduct', and Mrs Disney 'a most dangerous woman'.[6] Bracebridge wrote that Mrs Bessant, a 54-year-old widow with five years' experience at the London Hospital, was dismissed because of intoxication and being too old for the work. Mary Stanley, who was the most generous of the reference writers, crossed out 'intoxication' and wrote 'Mrs Bessant was a hard-working woman with whom I had no fault to find. She was sent home from Therapia on account of her health solely. Selena Bracebridge never saw her.'[7]

Despite these limitations, the references the five lady superintendents wrote indicate that they were practical, competent women who were prepared to accept the failings of their nurses if their nursing work was good. Nightingale expected the most, wanting the same complete commitment to the work as she herself had. However, unlike Bracebridge, Nightingale extended help and support to the women. Of the five lady superintendents, Nightingale's testimonials are the fullest; she kept good records of the women whom she paid, but she did not pay or even meet all of the nurses for whom we have documentation, and even she could leave out a name.

[3]   FNM/LMA/H01/ST/NC8/1; Summers, *Angels and Citizens*, pp. 40–42.

[4]   E. Davis, *The Autobiography of Elizabeth Davis, a Balaclava Nurse*, ed. J. Williams (London, 1857).

[5]   FNM/LMA/H01/ST/NC8/1, p. 15.

[6]   Ibid., pp. 9, 11.

[7]   Ibid., p. 11.

The memoir writers, the five lady superintendents and Elizabeth Davis all support each other to a surprising degree. The ladies would probably have completely agreed with Davis's analysis of the working-class nurses. Many, Davis wrote:

> were sent out as nurses who had never filled any place of trust before, and were really incapable of the duties which they had undertaken. Some among them, too, were persons of unsteady habits, who, not doing well at home, hoped to fare better abroad. Others were good women, and excellent nurses, and deserved to be trusted.

Davis classed herself in the last group.[8] Mother Francis Bridgeman described her as 'a hard working, honest old woman but quite a character, who did just what she pleased'.[9] Nightingale would undoubtedly have endorsed this portrayal. She characterized Davis as 'an active, respectable, hard-working, kind-hearted old woman with a foul tongue & a cross temper'. Nightingale said she would gladly have kept her till the end of the war, but Davis became ill and was invalided home in November 1855.[10] If the ladies' records are neither complete nor always consistently judged, they represent a watershed in the historiography of nursing because it is the first time we have first-hand information about hospital nurses from able women who actually worked with them. They tell us a very great deal about nursing in the 1850s.

The word 'nurse' had a different meaning from that of today, which makes it difficult for the modern reader to understand the nature of nursing in the mid-nineteenth century. We have seen how Golding used 'nurse' interchangeably with 'menial' in 1819. Kinglake, in his history of the Crimean War published in 1880, found it astounding that upper-class women were willing to do 'no more than "nurse" – simply "nurse" the poor sufferers',[11] an illustration of how unthinkable it was that ladies would do work which was considered menial. The fluid boundaries between domestic service and what we now call professional nursing were only just beginning to be drawn. As we have seen, most people saw hospital nurses as maids-of-all-work who cooked two of the patients' four daily meals, did a good deal of laundry, cleaned the patients, floors and furniture, and in addition gave some nursing care. Victorians used the term 'nurse' indiscriminately for women working in hospitals whether they actually delivered patient care, worked in hospital store rooms, or did the laundry, needlework, cooking and cleaning. The opposite also

---

[8]   Davis, *The Autobiography of Elizabeth Davis*, vol. 2, pp. 110–11.

[9]   Mother F. Bridgeman, 'An Account of the Mission of the Sisters of Mercy', in Maria Luddy (ed.), *The Crimean Journals of the Sisters of Mercy 1854–56* (Dublin, 2004), p. 196.

[10]   LMA/H01/ST/NC1/60/1.1–1.2; FNM/LMA/H1/St/NC8/1, p. 10.

[11]   A.W. Kinglake, *The Invasion of the Crimea: Its Origin and an Account of its Progress Down to the Death of Lord Raglan* (6 vols, New York, 1880), vol. 4, pp. 280–81.

occurred, as when Elizabeth Davis referred to the highly accomplished nurse Eliza Roberts as Nightingale's 'maid'.[12]

The arrangements for the cooking and the laundry in the army hospitals make it even harder for us now to understand the nature of military nursing during the Crimean War. The army's hospital kitchens prepared a number of simple diets which varied somewhat according to the doctor in charge, but usually the daily ration for a full diet was one pound of meat, one pound of potatoes, two pints of tea, and a half pint of porter. Then the doctors ordered 'extras' for individual patients. The nurses cooked the extras, which consisted of stimulants such as wine and brandy, and food such as chicken, mutton chops, milk, eggs, arrowroot, rice, sago or lemonade, in what were called their 'extra diet kitchens'.[13] As a result, the nurses spent a great deal of their time cooking. The matrons in the London hospitals had originally been housekeepers for whom the linen store was a major part of their work, so much so that they were often promoted from charge of the linen room to matron.[14] When the first party of nurses arrived in Scutari, there were no sheets or shirts. The soldiers had only the shirts on their backs when they came into the hospital, and they were incredibly filthy. With 2,000 men in the two hospitals, in November only six shirts were washed.[15] Supplying sheets, shirts and laundering and mending them therefore became a major part of the nurses' work.

As a result of the different kind of work which the nurses did in the 1850s, there are women whom the lady nurses classified as 'hospital nurses' who never dealt with patients. Mrs Suter was the cook at the Smyrna Hospital. Mary Viney had had some training at the Middlesex Hospital, but worked in the laundry. Martha Eskip, a 40-year-old widow, was a patient for six weeks at the Middlesex Hospital, and was then hired by the hospital as a nurse; in Scutari she was a laundress.[16] On the other hand, Elizabeth Davis was an experienced accident ward nurse from Guy's Hospital, but spent most of her time at the Balaclava General Hospital as the cook.[17] Sister Mary Aloysius Doyle was considered the best nurse among Mother Francis Bridgeman's 14 Sisters who were all accomplished nurses, but when Davis was invalided home, Bridgeman sent Doyle to the kitchen as her replacement.[18]

[12]   Davis, *The Autobiography of Elizabeth Davis*, vol. 2, pp. 117, 183–4.

[13]   F.M. Taylor, *Eastern Hospitals and English Nurses: The Narrative of Twelve Months Experience in the Hospitals of Koulali and Scutari* (1st edn, 2 vols, London, 1856), vol. 1, pp. 74, 78.

[14]   LMA/H09/GY/D40/1, pp. 1–3.

[15]   *PP*, 1854–55, vol. 9, Part 1, pp. 20, 674; ibid., Part 2, p. 21.

[16]   LMA/H01/ST/NC8/1, pp. 17, 27, 32; BL 43402, fol. 17.

[17]   Davis, *The Autobiography of Elizabeth Davis*, vol. 2, pp. 126–9, 134–5.

[18]   F. Taylor, *Eastern Hospitals and English Nurses* (3rd edn, London, 1857), pp. 319–22.

### The Lady Nurses: Kind Intentions, a Strong Constitution but a Lack of Clinical Experience

The nurses were a heterogeneous group: the majority were working-class, but there were some middle-class ladies, and even two minor aristocrats.[19] They can be classified into four groups: 128 working-class women, 9 Anglican Sisters, 28 Catholic Sisters and 50 ladies, plus Nightingale and Mary Stanley – a total of 217.[20] There were inefficient nurses among all four groups, but Nightingale found the volunteer secular ladies the least satisfactory and the hardest to work with. Nearly all had spent no more than a few days, or at most two or three weeks, training in hospitals, a totally inadequate period to become a competent clinical nurse in the 1850s. Furthermore, ladies were not used to the discipline required in a hospital nor to taking orders from other ladies.[21] Securing compliance with authority from a number of the ladies became one of Nightingale's biggest trials. Many lady nurses were not interested in establishing the extra diet kitchens, finding the soldiers furniture and clothing and setting up laundries and bath houses, which became Nightingale's primary concerns. They preferred nursing individual patients, which Nightingale characterized as 'pottering & messing about with little cookeries of individual Beef Teas for the poor sufferers personally'.[22]

A small number of the ladies were complete disasters. Mary Stanley, a personal friend of Nightingale's, was by far the most difficult. Stanley, who arrived in Scutari with 47 women in December 1854, believed Sidney Herbert wanted her and her party to report not to Nightingale, but to Dr Cumming, the principal medical officer at the Barrack Hospital.[23] Herbert later denied this,[24] but Stanley steadfastly refused to acknowledge Nightingale's authority, while at the same time she expected Nightingale to finance and make all the arrangements for her group.[25] Stanley had no clinical nursing experience, and her concept of nursing was based on the old view of sickness as a result of sin. She had visited many hospitals, and had just published a little book, *Hospitals and Sisterhoods*, in which she argued that the major problem in English hospitals was the paucity of chaplains.[26] She therefore wanted all lady nurses, whom she planned to use not as nurses, but as assistants to the chaplains and priests. This infuriated Nightingale, who appreciated

[19]   LMA/H01/ST/NC8/1. These two ladies were Jane Shaw Stewart and the Honorable Harriet Erskine.

[20]   LMA/H01/ST/NC8/1; WI/Ms/8997/11.

[21]   Summers, *Angels and Citizens*, p. 3.

[22]   BL Add Mss 43393, fols 147–8.

[23]   See, for example, BL 43393, fols 192–203.

[24]   A. H.-G. Stanmore, *Sidney Herbert, Lord Herbert of Lea: A Memoir* (2 vols, London, 1906), vol. 1, pp. 412–16. See also S. Goldie (ed.), *Florence Nightingale: Letters from the Crimea 1854–56* (Manchester, 1997), p. 50.

[25]   BL 43393, fols 142–5, 155–6.

[26]   M. Stanley, *Hospitals and Sisterhoods* (London, 1854), pp. 1–2, 10–28.

that clinical experience was essential for an effective nurse. Nevertheless, when the Koulali hospitals opened in late January 1855, Nightingale thought Stanley the best-qualified of those available to serve as superintendent.[27]

Charlotte Salisbury, a former governess in the family of the British consul at Patras, Greece, was the most disastrous of the lady nurses. She never nursed in the sense of giving patient care, but was hired in May 1855 to work with Selena Bracebridge in the Free Gifts Store, which consisted of the numerous gifts which private citizens sent out for the soldiers. When the Bracebridges left three months later, Salisbury took charge. No sooner were the Bracebridges gone than Salisbury began stealing from the gifts, and even from Nightingale herself. When Nightingale dismissed her in October 1855, she returned to London, where, with the help of Mary Stanley and others – largely nurses whom Nightingale had dismissed – she launched a libel suit against Nightingale. Elizabeth Davis joined this group, and without mentioning the source, incorporated in her autobiography the whole of Salisbury's untruthful statement in her own defence. The suit ultimately failed because investigations incontrovertibly showed that she and several accomplices had indeed stolen huge amounts of goods.[28]

Nightingale also dismissed Martha Clough, another lady with no hospital experience whom Nightingale described as an adventurer. Mother Emma Langston, superintendent of the Balaclava General Hospital where Clough worked, asked Nightingale to dismiss her because she encouraged drinking and insubordination among the working-class nurses. Nightingale later learned that when Clough first arrived in Turkey, she had taken three working-class nurses out drinking in a spirit shop. Clough claimed she had come out with the nursing team as a means of getting to Bulgaria to visit the grave of Lieutenant Colonel Lauderdale Maule, who had died there in August 1854. It is not certain what Clough's relationship to Maule was, but she said she 'had loved, honoured and appreciated him for nearly twenty long years'. In March 1855, Clough left Langston's team without informing Nightingale and took charge of Sir Colin Campbell's Highlanders' regimental hospital. She never got to Bulgaria, for in August 1855 she contracted fever, and died the following month.[29]

Altogether, six lady nurses were discharged: the two above by Nightingale, and four by Henrietta LeMesurier. LeMesurier dismissed Miss Tomlinson because she thought she was insane, Miss Jackson because she was 'unsuitable in every way', Miss Winthrop because she was a mischievous person who spread evil reports and was on bad terms with the other ladies, and Mrs Brereton because she showed

---

[27]   BL 43393, fols 46, 148–9.

[28]   I.B. O'Malley, *Florence Nightingale 1820–1856: A Study of Her Life Down to the End of the Crimean War* (London, 1934), pp. 321–8; LMA/H01/ST/NC1/60/1.1–1.2; WI/Ms/8995/56.

[29]   National Library of Scotland GD/45/9/337/1–12; BL 43397 fol. 207; Sir R. Roxburgh, 'Miss Nightingale and Miss Clough', *Victorian Studies*, 13/1 (1969): pp. 71–2, 87–8.

'a great want of discretion and most discreditable disorder in her preliminary negotiations'.[30]

There were some ladies who, Nightingale thought, were not competent to superintend, but whom she nevertheless promoted because superintendents had to be literate and the Victorian class system decreed that only ladies had the status and authority to direct working-class women. Elizabeth Davis accepted this convention. She believed ladies should not perform the 'servile offices' of a nurse. By so doing, they 'hurt the feelings of the men [soldiers], who were acutely sensible of the unfitness of such work for persons of high station. Ladies may be fit to govern,' Davis wrote, but working-class nurses were more useful as nurses.[31] Sister Mary Aloysius Doyle took a more practical view. The secular lady nurses, she said, '*admit they know nothing about nursing*, many of them never having seen a dead person'. They therefore depended heavily on the religious Sisters. '*How could they superintend without some knowledge of the work*,' Doyle asked; '*This they admitted and regretted.*'[32]

Miss Margaret Wear is one example of a lady superintendent who was appointed simply because she was a lady. The daughter of a lawyer, she had been living abroad for 17 years, and claimed she had trained in foreign hospitals.[33] Nightingale needed a superintendent for the Koulali hospitals because Mary Stanley planned to leave in the spring, so she sent Wear to Koulali on trial. After only one day, Stanley decided she was entirely unsuitable and sent her back. Nightingale herself thought Wear 'too eccentric to be of any use', and placed her in the Scutari General Hospital as a nurse, not a superintendent. However, in April 1855, when Jane Shaw Stewart, the superintendent of the Balaclava General Hospital, left to become superintendent of the newly opened Castle Hospital, having no better lady to replace her, Nightingale sent Wear.[34]

Wear is an illustration of a nurse who did not have nursing expertise, but whom her patients liked because of her kindnesses – she pottered and messed about with individual patients, as Nightingale put it. Wear worked incredible hours, sometimes doing night duty six nights out of seven. She gave the same care and attention to the French, Sardinians and Russians,[35] whether officers or men. Every morning

---

[30]    FNM/LMA/H1/ST/NC8/1, pp. 12–14.

[31]    Davis, *The Autobiography of Elizabeth Davis*, vol. 2, p. 137. In fact, the soldiers were not embarrassed by the lady nurses. As one sergeant reported: 'There was no sort of delicacy about them'; M.H. Mawson (ed.), *Eyewitness in the Crimea: The Crimean War Letters 1854–1856 of Lt. Col. George Frederick Dallas* (London, 2001), p. 59.

[32]    Sister M.A. Doyle, 'Memories of the Crimea', in Luddy (ed.), *The Crimean Journals of the Sisters of Mercy*, pp. 27–8 (original emphases).

[33]    FNM/LMA/H1/ST/NC8/1, p. 14.

[34]    BL 43396, fols 30–31; FNM/LMA/H1/ST/NC8/1, p. 14.

[35]    The English, French and Turks were fighting the Russians. The Sardinians joined the allies in January 1855. Their troops arrived in Balaclava on 8 May 1855; Baumgart, *The Crimean War 1853–56*, p. 89.

she went through the wards to see that the orderlies had put everything the patients needed within their reach, and she gave the men many 'extras'. She helped in the kitchen, and because she spoke French and Italian, was very useful as an interpreter. When Nightingale told Dr John Hall, the English chief medical officer, that she was not satisfied with Wear's superintending and suggested replacing her, Hall strongly supported Wear. Among other things, he liked her treatment of the Sardinian officers. Even so, Wear's arrangements at the Balaclava hospital did not follow Nightingale's system, and Mother Francis Bridgeman, a highly experienced and competent nurse, was appalled by the state in which she found parts of the hospital when she arrived there in October 1855. Bridgeman thought Elizabeth Davis's kitchen, under Wear's supervision, 'the most discreditable establishment one could well imagine … with filth and disorder everywhere'.[36]

After the government sent dressers to the hospitals at the end of December 1854, the nurses were no longer allowed to do dressings. As well, with the arrival of Mary Stanley's large group of women, there were twice as many nurses as there had been in November and most of December. Nightingale therefore asked her superintendents to avoid caring for individual patients, but rather to concentrate on superintendence and sound financial practice. She felt Wear spent too much time personally nursing individual patients, and not enough time on supervision. Wear also seems to have lost large amounts of the supplies which Nightingale sent for the General and Castle Hospitals. Nightingale thought she was not basically dishonest, but simply too un-businesslike to keep good records.[37] Another indication of Wear's incompetence as a superintendent is that she, more than anyone else, including the suspicious Selena Bracebridge, accused nurses, including Elizabeth Woodward who was a model nurse, of being impertinent to her and exhibiting 'violent and unruly conduct' towards her.[38] Finally, like Clough and Stanley, Wear decided she would not take orders from Nightingale. She began working directly for Hall.[39]

Another lady superintendent, Mrs Willoughby Moore, was an older woman, the widow of an officer who died when his ship sank on its way to the Crimea.[40] She came with two nurses and her maid to set up the Palace Hospital, thus named because it was the Sultan's summer palace which he had donated for a hospital for officers. Less than two months after arriving, in November 1855, Willoughby Moore died of fever. Nightingale believed: 'She killed herself by going out boating at night with the officers she was sent to nurse.'[41]

---

[36]    Davis, *The Autobiography of Elizabeth Davis*, vol. 2, pp. 150–51, 156–7, 174; Bridgeman, 'Mission of the Sisters', p. 196.

[37]    BL 43393, fol. 64; BL 39867, fols 71–2; WI/Ms/8995/69.

[38]    LMA/H01/ST/NC8/1, p.7; V. Bonham-Carter (ed.), *Surgeon in the Crimea: The Experiences of George Lawson* (London, 1968), pp. 175, 179–80, 193–4 n. 9.

[39]    BL 39867, fols 34, 37–8, 63.

[40]    WI/Ms/8895/26.

[41]    Wiltshire County Record Office/2057/F4/68.

Few ladies were used to the hard physical work which hospital nursing entailed, while others were too old to start. Mrs Lloyd Jones, a 50-year-old officer's widow who spent ten weeks in training in Guy's Hospital, came with high testimonials, but was invalided home because she was too old for the work. Misses Osborne, Aplin and Piper were excellent persons, but also not strong enough for the work.[42] In the analysis of Sister Mary Aloysius Doyle, because the ladies came from luxurious homes they were totally physically unfit for the arduous work of acute care nursing. Trained in a novitiate of four and a half years, Doyle was, by contrast, both clinically expert and accustomed to the heavy physical demands of nursing.[43]

Other ladies were acceptable, but had some major failing. Mrs Annabella McLeod and her daughter Abigail were two of the seven paid lady nurses. McLeod, the 51-year-old widow of an army officer, was in charge of the Nurses' Home at Koulali. When those hospitals closed, she and Abigail went to Scutari, where Nightingale had them help with the linen stores and supervise the seamstresses. McLeod was most amiable and attractive, but she was so old and in such delicate health that she could not do any serious work. The ladies thought Abigail excellent, full of courage and energy, but not 'useful',[44] by which they probably meant she was not prepared to do the drudging work.

Miss Tebbutt, the matron of the Scutari General Hospital, had more serious failings. Nightingale thought her entirely unfitted to be a superintendent, and even less to be a nurse, but she appreciated Tebbutt's care of the nurses' morals, which indeed was an important part of the job in the 1850s. After Charlotte Salisbury mounted the libel case against Nightingale, Mary Stanley, whose judgement seemed to be singularly lacking in this area, kept in touch with Tebbutt, who sometimes lied to keep Stanley's letters from Nightingale, while at other times she showed them to her. In one letter, Stanley covertly accused Selena Bracebridge and Nightingale of falsehood and theft. Nightingale could hardly believe that Tebbutt would have credited such accusations. She considered Tebbutt 'a weak fool' who lacked common sense. Still, Tebbutt seems to have been well liked by her colleagues, and even more so by Chaplain Hadow, who proposed to her. She did not accept him, which was a strike in her favour in Nightingale's view, for she did not have a high opinion of Hadow. In November 1855, when the Koulali and Smyrna Hospitals closed, Nightingale tried unsuccessfully to replace Tebbutt with one of the ladies from those two hospitals.[45]

Ten of the secular ladies were excellent workers, and three of those ten, Anne Ward Morton, Mary Tattersall and Jane Shaw Stewart, positively superb. However, because none, with the exception of Shaw Stewart, had any real experience

---

[42]  FNM/LMA/H1/ST/NC8/1, pp. 12, 15.

[43]  Doyle, 'Memories of the Crimea', pp. 27–8.

[44]  FNM/LMA/H01/ST/NC8/1, p. 24, BL 43402, fol. 10.

[45]  BL 43402, fol. 16; BL 45792, fols 61–2; WI/Mss/8996/28 and 69; S. Terrot, *Reminiscences of Scutari Hospitals in Winter 1854–55* (Edinburgh, 1898), p. 80; FNM/ H01/ST/NC8/1, p. 7.

with modern hospital nursing practice, Nightingale used them largely as matrons or housekeepers. By contrast, before leaving for Turkey, Shaw Stewart had spent a number of weeks in training at the Westminster and Guy's.[46] Many ladies only observed in the hospitals, but she apparently actually nursed. She became one of Nightingale's main supports during the war years, although Nightingale thought her 'unwise, provoking and mad'. Nightingale was not exaggerating. George Lawson, a young army surgeon, thought her 'perfectly mad'. She sat up almost every night with her fever patients, and slept, wrapped in her cloak, on the ground. A young cavalry officer, Temple Godman, thought her '*quite* cracked' and very odd. But 'mad as she is', Nightingale wrote, she was 'above mean, petty, selfish and frivolous behaviour'.[47]

Shaw Stewart's mental instability became even more obvious after the war. At St John's House, where Nightingale sent her for further training, Sister Mary Jones found her extremely uncooperative.[48] Later, as superintendent of Netley Hospital, she flew into passions, stamping her feet, slamming doors, talking very loudly, physically beating the nurses, sending lengthy letters and memoranda to the medical staff and snapping her fingers in their faces. Not surprisingly, she was unable to keep her staff. After one of her encounters with a doctor, she announced that if she could not enter the wards with authority, she would blow up the nurses' quarters. This behaviour led to her dismissal in 1868.[49]

During the war, however, Shaw Stewart's aristocratic connections, her bearing and her total commitment to nursing the soldiers commanded respect from all the other nurses. Even the difficult Martha Clough esteemed her highly, while Elizabeth Davis felt she was the only lady in the East who was really a competent nurse. Davis considered her 'odd' at times, but just and firm, and thought that under her direction, the Crimean hospitals finally began to work well. Davis described how she followed her out at night in the dark, 'through the bad weather and along the worst roads possible, to visit the sick and wounded, and to carry lemonade and other drinks from our kitchen to the huts'.[50] Nightingale made Shaw Stewart successively superintendent of the General, Castle and Left Wing Land Transport Corps Hospitals.[51]

Anne Ward Morton was the sister of a University College Hospital doctor, had nursed cholera patients as a district visitor, and trained briefly at the Westminster Hospital. She was matron of the Barrack Hospital, and later took charge of the linen

---

[46]   LMA/H02/WH/A1/37, 24 October, 5 December 1854; Summers, *Angels and Citizens*, p. 42.

[47]   BL 45793, fol. 106; Bonham-Carter, *Surgeon in the Crimea*, p. 164; P. Warner (ed.), *The Fields of War: A Young Cavalryman's Crimea Campaign* (London, 1977), pp. 139–40 (original emphasis); WI/Ms/8995/56.

[48]   BL 47743, fols 98–102.

[49]   BL 45774, fols 102–06.

[50]   Davis, *The Autobiography of Elizabeth Davis*, vol. 2, pp. 137–8. The Balaclava General Hospital consisted of a stone building containing seven wards plus 14 separate huts.

[51]   WI/Ms/8997/58.

stores. In the evenings she taught the nurses reading and writing, helping to 'raise their characters'. Morton was willing to take any work which needed to be done, but she lacked physical strength, which prevented her doing as much as she would have liked.[52]

Mary Tattersall was the daughter of a Leeds brewer, and was one of the paid lady nurses. She had been a district visitor, and then trained for three weeks at the Westminster before going to Scutari. On receiving her first pay, she sent the Westminster £5. She wanted to donate some of the first money she ever earned, she said, to the hospital where she received so much kindness as a student. Tattersall's untiring industry, her flinching from no menial employment, 'her truth, judgement, faithfulness, discretion & entire trustworthiness, her temperance in all things, even in flirting, & her high religious principles' earned Nightingale's respect and esteem. Nevertheless, Nightingale did not use her for patient care, but as cook and housekeeper for the female staff of the Scutari General Hospital.[53]

Morton and Tattersall – both excellent workers, but in areas other than patient care – illustrate how important clinical experience and familiarity with modern medical practice had become. Only Jane Shaw Stewart nursed in the sense of giving patient care. It was also obvious that hospital nurses required robust health and the strength gained from a life of hard work. The Crimean War experience seemed to suggest that as long as ladies maintained their relative monopoly on education and the lower classes continued to respect their social status and authority, the secular ladies' future role in nursing would be as old-style housekeeper matrons.

**The Religious Nurses: Nursing Expertise, Religious Discipline and Administrative Skills**

*The Anglican Sisters*

Three Anglican Sisters from the Park Village Sisterhood and five from Priscilla Lydia Sellon's Devonport Sisters of Mercy[54] accompanied Nightingale to Scutari in October 1854. As the Superior of the Park Village Sisterhood, Mother Emma Langston had not been a success, but because of her seniority she was placed in charge of the other seven Sisters. While her own Sisters thought she was an excellent nurse, Nightingale claimed her patients were cruelly neglected and had bed sores. Nightingale also feared Langton was slipping into senility. She was niggling and tiresome about trifles, and continually wishing for a situation where she could do

[52]    WI/Mss/8995/65, 68 and 79; FNM/LMA/H1/ST/NC8/1, p. 38; BL 43402, fol. 25.

[53]    FNM/LMA/H1/ST/NC8/1, p. 23; 8995/79; WI/Ms/8996/69; J.C. Humble and P. Hansell, *Westminster Hospital 1716–1966* (London, 1966), p. 81; BL 43402, fol. 16.

[54]    To disassociate herself from the much-maligned and disliked High Church position of these two sisterhoods, Nightingale always publicly referred to them as 'Sellonites', but her contemporaries did not use this term.

more, while unable to do the work she already had. She was invalided home in April 1855.[55] Sister Etheldreda Pillans had been so seasick on the voyage out that on arrival in Scutari, she was too weak to do any work. Nightingale sent her home immediately.[56] The third Park Village Sister, the Honourable Harriet Mary Erskine, was a 'certificated nurse'. By the 1890s this term meant someone who had spent two or three years working in a hospital with a certain amount of instruction, but in 1854 it usually meant someone who had spent perhaps a few weeks in a hospital, largely unsupervised, and often only observing. Selena Bracebridge thought that, although willing and obedient, Erskine was not much of a nurse. She was invalided home at the end of April 1855, but later came back to Turkey as a superintendent of the naval hospital in Therapia.[57]

The Devonport Sisters all had considerable nursing experience, having nursed during the cholera epidemics of 1849 and 1853. In the 1849 epidemic they ran a temporary hospital with two marquees, one for the Sisters and one for children orphaned by the disease.[58] Sister Sarah Anne Terrot, a daughter of the Bishop of Edinburgh, had nursed in both cholera epidemics. She was conscientious, single-purposed, never refused any work or asked for more than she could do, but Nightingale considered her neither clever nor efficient. Still, Nightingale appreciated her 'disinterested, unambitious work'. Terrot was invalided home in April 1855.[59] Child[60] Clara Sharpe had been in charge of the Sisters' small hospital in Bristol. Nightingale thought she was good and gentle, but awkward on account of her hands. It is not clear what the problem with her hands was, but Terrot agreed that they disqualified her from military nursing. She was sent home in December 1854.[61]

Sister Bertha Turnbull and Novice Margaret Goodman[62] were two of the few nurses, ladies or working-class, who never fell ill and so worked the whole nineteen months till the end of the war. They attributed this to having followed Mother Superior Sellon's instructions to take an hour of recreation every day,

[55]   PHA, Nightingale to Sellon, 5 December 1854; T.J. Williams and A.W. Campbell, *The Park Village Sisterhood* (London, 1965), pp. 24–5, 89–90; WI/Ms/8995/78.

[56]   Williams and Campbell, *The Park Village Sisterhood*, p. 96; WI/Ms/8995/78.

[57]   BUNA, Nightingale Collection/2/3/B2; FNM/LMA/H1/ST/NC8/1, p. 2; WI/Ms 5482/14; C. Lloyd and J.L.S. Coulter (eds), *Medicine and the Navy 1200–1900* (4 vols, Edinburgh, 1963), vol. 4, p. 149.

[58]   T.J. Williams, *Priscilla Lydia Sellon: The Restorer after Three Centuries of the Religious Life in the English Church* (London, 1950), pp. 71–5, 136.

[59]   PHA, Nightingale to Sellon, 5 December 1854 and 5 March 1855, FNM/LMA/H1/ ST/NC8/1, p. 2.

[60]   The Devonport Sisters had unusual titles. 'Child' was the equivalent of a postulant, a candidate for admission to a religious order who has not yet been admitted as a novice.

[61]   PHA, Nightingale to Sellon, 5 December 1854; Williams, *Priscilla Lydia Sellon*, p. 135; WI/Ms/8995/78.

[62]   Margaret Goodman's official status and title was actually Child Margaret. She is sometimes called Sister or Lay Sister Margaret, and at other times Novice Margaret.

usually walking out in the fresh air.[63] Turnbull was the daughter of an Edinburgh chamberlain, a position roughly equivalent to a city treasurer. At first, Nightingale considered her 'the steadiest and fittest for command' of the nurses. She later reversed her opinion, but then changed her mind yet again, deciding she had 'first rate qualities of head and heart'. When Jane Shaw Stewart left the Castle Hospital to become superintendent of a wing of the Land Transport Hospital, Nightingale replaced her with Turnbull. Nightingale thought she did not have such commanding abilities as Shaw Stewart – after all, she was not an aristocrat – but she was a first-class nurse, faithful and devoted, who always showed excellent judgement. All the soldiers who had heard of her loved her.[64] Nightingale later felt it unfair that she received all the acclaim for the work in the Crimean War when others such as Turnbull had contributed so much.[65]

Margaret Goodman was a farmer's daughter, and had been a primary schoolmistress before joining the Devonport Sisters in 1852. She taught in the sisterhood's schools and nursed during the 1853 cholera epidemic. She was well educated, knew French, played the piano and organ, and led the singing at the Sunday evening services in the Scutari General Hospital. Nightingale thought her 'as valuable as Sister Bertha in her different sphere & different duties, an excellent nurse and perfectly above all or any wishes but that of doing her duty.'[66]

The one Anglican Sister with whom Nightingale had difficulty was Sister Elizabeth Wheeler. The sister of an Anglican clergyman, she impressed Nightingale with her commanding and stately presence at first, but Nightingale quickly changed her mind. One of the first things Wheeler told Nightingale was that she hoped the Sisters would be treated as ladies, and indeed some of the Sisters expected a great deal of waiting on; they were not used to cleaning up or to what Nightingale called drudging, and at first it took one nurse her whole shift to clean up after them. The working-class nurses disliked Wheeler intensely, but the other Devonport Sisters were devoted to her, while her patients loved her cheerful, frank and gentle manner.[67]

The doctors in charge of Wheeler's wards ordered a great many extras for the men, but even when available, which they often were not in November and December 1854, extras were always in short supply. Wheeler tried to get preferential treatment for her patients, and constantly complained about the shortages to Nightingale, ignoring the fact that no ward had enough food, or for that matter,

---

[63]    Williams, *Priscilla Lydia Sellon*, pp. 176–7.

[64]    PHA, Nightingale to Sellon, 5 December 1854; FNM/H1/ST/NC8/1, p. 2; BL 43402, fol. 21; WI/Ms/8997/58.

[65]    Nightingale to Mary Shore Smith, 30 July 1888, Private Collection of Hugh Small.

[66]    BL 43402, fol. 21; WI/Ms/8997/58; LMA/H01/ST/NC2/V1/59.

[67]    PHA, Nightingale to Mother Priscilla Lydia Sellon, 5 December 1854; Terrot, *Reminiscences of Scutari Hospitals*, pp. 28–9.

enough shirts or other supplies.[68] Further difficulties arose when Wheeler wrote to a relative asking him to send food and wine for the patients. The government has not been remiss, she wrote, but there were so many wounded that it was impossible to meet their wants. The relative sent the letter to *The Times*, which published it on 29 November 1854.[69] Nightingale had been sent to Scutari to appease the outcry against the failings of the army's medical and supply system;[70] Wheeler's letter fed that uproar and enraged the army doctors. On 23 December a commission of three doctors and a lawyer cross-examined Sister Elizabeth, trying to get her to admit that she had lied. Because she was a woman, even though a lady, they treated her much as the Middlesex governors had Cookesley: they did not give her a copy of the letter, and did not tell her which statements they considered untrue. She became confused and appeared to prevaricate. The commission pronounced her letter inaccurate and contradictory to her oral evidence, and tried to make her confess that she was guilty of lying. They even threatened her with penal consequences if she did not sign a confession which they had written. Wheeler refused to sign because she did not believe she had told any untruth. The commission decided she should be dismissed immediately, and Nightingale, who had given evidence against her, ruthlessly complied.[71]

A ninth Sister, Sister Anne Thom from the Park Village Sisterhood, arrived in March 1855. She was the sister of a doctor and a clergyman in Aberdeenshire, and had been a surgical nurse at the Middlesex, where she was highly esteemed. The superintendents at Koulali, where she worked, found her very sensible and skilful. She was much and deservedly admired by both patients and orderlies, and it was she who introduced night nursing at Koulali. When, in November 1855, the doctors insisted that the diet orders be strictly enforced and that the ladies could no longer give extras on their own authority, one of the lady nurses said the ladies did not know what to do with themselves. Four lady nurses and Miss Hutton, the superintendent, resigned. Thom was then put in charge. Nightingale accepted nurses at Scutari from other hospitals which were closing if they were willing to accept her stricter rules. Thom apparently was prepared to do this, but Nightingale recognized her nursing capacities and did not feel that she had a suitable opening for her. Thom returned to England on 21 December 1855.[72]

---

[68]   *PP*, 1854–55, vol. 9, Part 1, pp. 279–83; O'Malley, *Florence Nightingale*, pp. 240, 246–7, Terrot, *Reminiscences of Scutari Hospitals*, pp. 44–5.

[69]   PHA, article cut from *The Times*, 29 November 1854.

[70]   C. Helmstadter, 'Navigating the Straits of the Crimean War', in S. Nelson and A.M. Rafferty (eds), *Notes on Nightingale* (Ithaca, NY, 2010), pp. 29–30.

[71]   *PP*, 1854–55, vol. 33, pp. 329–31; Terrot, *Reminiscences of Scutari Hospitals*, pp. 11, 28–9, 44–5, 73–5; O'Malley, *Florence Nightingale*, p. 260.

[72]   FNM/LMA/H1/ST/ NC8/1, p. 20; Taylor, *Eastern Hospitals and English Nurses*, 1st edn, vol. 1, pp. 224–6; ibid., vol. 2, pp. 171–3, 254, 256, 263.

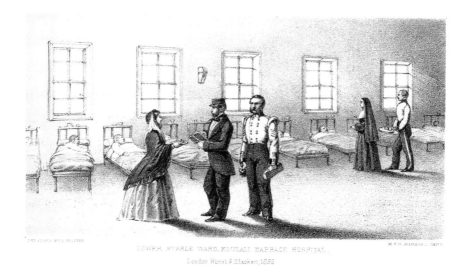

LOWER STABLE WARD, KOULALI BARRACK HOSPITAL.

London Hurst & Blackett, 1856

Figure 5.1    The Koulali Lower Hospital, 1855. A lady nurse who is officially in charge takes orders from the surgeon and his assistant, while in the background a nun and an orderly give patient care. The artist, who was one of the soldiers, did not include a working-class nurse in the scene.

*Source*: Wellcome Library, London, by kind permission.

*The Catholic Sisters*

Three different groups of Roman Catholic Sisters served in the war. The first group, five nuns from the Convent of Our Lady of the Orphans in Norwood, were sent home in December 1854 because they came from an enclosed order and had no hospital nursing experience.[73] The second party, the Bermondsey Sisters, were eminently successful, with their Mother Superior, Mary Clare Moore, becoming one of Nightingale's main supports. The third group, Mother Francis Bridgeman's party, proved unable to co-operate in the larger nursing project.

Moore's superlative administrative and accounting abilities were invaluable, so despite her excellent nursing skills, Nightingale soon put her in charge of the extra diet kitchen. Later, Moore took over the linen stores, where in May 1855, when the Scutari hospitals were much less crowded than in the preceding winter, she had to provide 1,000 shirts and 1,000 sheets weekly – an enormous job, but one which she managed efficiently. Nightingale feared losing public support if she placed a Catholic officially in charge of the hospital, so on her third trip to the

[73]    FNM/LMA/H01/ST/NC8/1, pp. 3–4; BA, pp. 231–2.

Crimea in the spring of 1856, Nightingale placed her aunt, Mai Smith, officially in charge of the Scutari hospitals. However, behind the scenes it was Moore who showed Smith how to run them. Nightingale considered Moore far above her 'in worldly talent of administration & far more in spiritual qualifications'.[74]

The other four Bermondsey Sisters were extraordinarily competent and experienced nurses. In December, Nightingale sent two, Sisters Jean de Chantal and Mary de Gonzaga, and Sisters Bertha, Margaret and Sarah Anne with ten working-class nurses to the Scutari General Hospital. Although wary of placing a Catholic formally in charge, she gave Gonzaga 'general charge' of the nurses for a short time. Sister Sarah Anne Terrot thought Gonzaga considerate and tactful, exercising her authority gently and wisely. Terrot commented: 'However much they [the Bermondsey Sisters] may have erred in faith and practice, their patient, gentle, cheerful manners and their constant kindness demonstrated a true and practical Christianity.' Nightingale did not write references for Moore and Gonzaga, but of the other three Sisters she said: 'Their faithfulness, their spirit, energy, true discernment of the right in many difficult, trying & vexed questions, their judgment, devotion, zeal and accuracy, – their cheerful resignation to inevitable opposition & enmity, have made them among our most valuable allies.'[75]

The Bermondsey Sisters were so successful that Nightingale requested three more. In late 1854, the convent had arranged for special training at St George's Hospital for Sisters who might later be sent to Scutari. Sisters Helen, Mary Joseph and Mary Martha arrived in November 1855, and eventually went to the Crimea, where Nightingale at last felt secure enough to put a Catholic officially in charge, making Sister Helen superintendent of a wing of the Land Transport Corps Hospitals. Nightingale thought it 'impossible to estimate too highly the unwearied devotion, patience, & cheerfulness, the judgement and activity & the single heartedness' of these three Sisters.[76]

Mother Francis Bridgeman was another story. She refused to accept Nightingale's authority, partly because Nightingale was a secular and a Protestant, and partly because of Irish hatred of the English ascendancy. Although Bridgeman and Moore signed essentially the same contract agreeing to act principally as nurses and to work under Nightingale's direction, they received different instructions from their respective bishops. Moore's bishop, Bishop Grant, was an Englishman, and although Moore was Irish, she had been living in England for 15 years except for one short interval, and was well aware of its ferocious anti-Catholic feelings. Moore was extremely diplomatic, and she and Grant were anxious not to arouse further anti-Catholic antagonisms. They agreed she should adhere strictly to the contract and that she and her nuns would work primarily as nurses.[77]

[74]   BA/Annals, pp. 258–9, 294; BA/Nightingale Collection, fols 8–11, 21, 26.

[75]   Terrot, *Reminiscences of Scutari Hospitals*, pp. 44, 70–71; BL Add Mss 43402, fol. 22.

[76]   SGH/MBG, 6 December 1854; BL 43402, fol. 10.

[77]   BA/Annals, pp. 242–3; Luddy, *The Crimean Journals of the Sisters of Mercy*, p. xv.

Bridgeman, by contrast, had been instructed by her bishop, Bishop William Delaney of Cork, to remain in the nursing team as long as it was at all possible, with the one condition that she must maintain her Sisters as a community under her own direction. More important, Delaney told her that nursing was not to be her top priority. 'Your calling is from God, and principally for the salvation of souls, and you could not undertake the mere task of nurse tending unaccompanied by the higher functions of your order,' he wrote to Bridgeman. He advised submitting to acting as nurses for the corporal needs of the body for a short time, while working towards the higher end of saving souls. Bridgeman and her Sisters did what she called 'instructing' – advising, influencing, sympathizing and instructing the soldiers in religion – which Nightingale felt crossed the line into proselytizing, something which the government had strictly forbidden.[78]

Although nursing was not her top priority, and despite the generally belligerent attitude she took towards Nightingale, Bridgeman and her nuns were highly experienced, proficient nurses. They showed the same professional approach as the Bermondsey Sisters: from the time they arrived in London in October until they left for Scutari on 2 December, Bridgeman and another Sister went every day to St George's or another hospital to study English nursing practice.[79] Nightingale would accuse them of leaving the Balaclava General Hospital in a filthy state,[80] but that appears to have been an exaggeration. The doctors and the soldiers, and indeed the Protestant superintendent at the Koulali Hospitals, all thought highly of their nursing.[81] Moore, on whom Bridgeman looked down because she co-operated with Nightingale, would also attest to their competent nursing. They 'had been greatly beloved by the Soldiers', she wrote, and 'had laboured efficiently among them'.[82]

Because Bridgeman kept her community apart from the other nurses, including the Bermondsey Sisters of Mercy, we do not have systematic assessments of the individual Sisters' work. Fanny Taylor, one of the more experienced lady nurses, for she had spent considerable time nursing with the Devonport Sisters, said that the Sisters' long experience caring for the sick and the poor made them superior nurses. Bridgeman, Taylor wrote, 'had long experience in hospital work and

[78]    E. Bolster, *The Sisters of Mercy in the Crimean War* (Cork, 1964), p. 125; Doyle, 'Memories of the Crimea', pp. 44–5; Bridgeman, 'Mission of the Sisters', pp. 177–8; Taylor, *Eastern Hospitals and English Nurses*, 1st edn, vol. 1, pp. 5–6; WI/Ms/8995/26.

[79]    Bridgeman, 'Mission of the Sisters', p. 124.

[80]    WI/Ms/8996/48.

[81]    Doyle, 'Memories of the Crimea', pp. 20, 27–8, 38, 57; Bridgeman, 'Mission of the Sisters', pp. 177, 198–9.

[82]    Luddy, *The Crimean Journals of the Sisters of Mercy*, pp. xviii–xix; Sullivan, *The Friendship of Florence Nightingale and Mary Clare Moore*, p. 70.

possessed a skill and judgment in nursing attained by few'. Sister Mary Aloysius Doyle supported her view.[83]

## Conclusion

After the war, Nightingale named five nurses whom she considered her mainstays. The first four were ladies: three religious Sisters – Mother Mary Clare Moore, Sisters Bertha Turnbull and Margaret Goodman – and one secular, Jane Shaw Stewart.[84] This would help fuel the myth of Nightingale and her 'educated, trained and refined' lady nurses moving into the hospitals and, almost overnight, revolutionizing nursing.[85] The fixation on lady nurses, which so irritated Nightingale and which Sister Mary Jones would later call 'sickly, sentimental nonsense',[86] would preserve the hierarchical social structure of mid-nineteenth-century England as an outstanding feature of nursing well into the twentieth century. In fact, the secular lady nurses were the least successful clinical nurses because they were unused to hard physical work and they lacked the hospital experience which had become essential by the 1850s. Apart from Nightingale, only two of the 52 secular lady nurses, Nightingale and Jane Shaw Stewart, had some months of hospital nursing experience, and after the war, Shaw Stewart proved an utter disaster. Some secular ladies did make outstanding contributions, but it was as old-style matrons, in charge of the linen, needlework, extra diet kitchens and the discipline of the working-class nurses.

The religious Sisters had both clinical experience and religious discipline, which made them exceptionally valuable. The Bermondsey nuns and Anglican Sisters understood the need for obedience and co-operation, were interested primarily in the nursing rather than adventure or giving religious instruction, and they had the necessary administrative and financial skills developed from running their convents. 'Give me [hospital] nurses, with a very small admixture of experienced ladies and a larger one of English nuns for the army hospitals,' Nightingale wrote at the end of the war.[87] Later, she declared that volunteer *untrained* ladies who offered themselves as nurses were 'the greatest mischief in her experience'.[88]

Nightingale's fifth exemplary nurse, Eliza Roberts, was one of the working-class hospital nurses. We turn now to explore the characteristics of these nurses and what they tell us about the way nursing practice had changed by the 1850s.

---

[83]   Taylor, *Eastern Hospitals and English Nurses*, 1st edn, vol. 1, pp. 261–2; ibid., vol. 2, pp. 28–9; Doyle, 'Memories of the Crimea', p. 20.

[84]   Leeds District Archives/Canning/177/2/3.

[85]   L.L. Dock and I.M. Stewart, *A Short History of Nursing from the Earliest Times to the Present Day* (4th edn, New York, 1938), p. 126.

[86]   BL Add Mss 47744, fols 138–9.

[87]   BL Add Mss 43402, fol. 6.

[88]   BL Add Mss 45818, fol. 33.

# Chapter 6
# Nursing at the Crossroads, Part 2:
# Working-class Nurses in the Crimean War

Many of the working-class nurses who served in the British military hospitals during the Crimean War presented a challenge to the lady superintendents because, while they were extremely valuable as nurses, they did not meet Victorian standards of propriety. Some were indeed very respectable and highly disciplined, while many others could work well if closely supervised. However, at least 34, or about a quarter, were dismissed.

## Clinical Expertise and Impropriety

Drink was a major problem across all social classes in England in the 1850s, and was the failing for which the largest number of hospital nurses were dismissed. Nightingale discharged Mrs Wilson before she even disembarked at Constantinople because of her drinking problem. Wilson had arrived drunk to join the first group of nurses when they left London Bridge Station on 19 October. The station master therefore turned her away. She then went to Nightingale's family, who gave her money which she spent travelling first-class to Marseilles, where she joined Nightingale's group. She announced publicly that she did not come out for the paltry 10s. a week, but to nurse noblemen; she planned to desert at the first opportunity.[1] Mary Stanley sent Nurses Anderson and Hefferman home immediately because they had also been drunk on the voyage out.

Many women whom the lady superintendents dismissed were excellent nurses, but had some serious failing, of which drink was the most common. A. Faulkner was a very good surgical nurse from the Royal Free Hospital, but she drank to excess. In addition, she had set herself up in business buying and selling things for the patients,[2] a fairly common practice among the old nurses, but one which hospital administrators decried. Martha Wheatstone was a very experienced nurse who had worked in three London hospitals: the Children's Hospital, the Royal Free and the Middlesex. She was a confirmed alcoholic, but otherwise a very valuable nurse. When Nightingale finally dismissed her for drunkenness in November 1855, Wheatstone returned to

---

[1]  WI/Ms/8894/115.

[2]  FNM/LMA/H1/ST/NC8/1, p. 4; WI/Ms/8995/78.

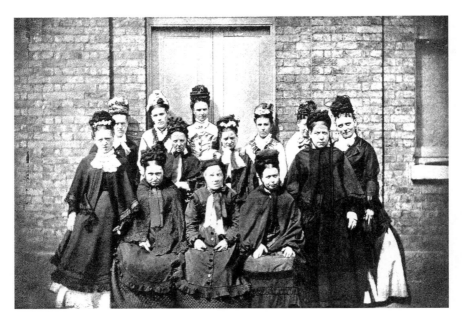

Figure 6.1     A group of Guy's nurses, *c.* 1860. This photograph, taken only
               a few years after the Crimean War, illustrates the different kinds
               and ages of the working-class women who traditionally went into
               nursing. These are not the nurses' working clothes, but rather their
               best clothes. They had two hours off in the evening every other day,
               when they could go out, and they are perhaps ready to set off for the
               pubs.

*Source*: Wellcome Library, London, by kind permission.


England and gave evidence against Nightingale in Salisbury's libel suit. Even so,
Nightingale was distressed to lose her excellent nursing skills.[3]

   Mrs Disney, Mrs Gibson and Mrs Whitehead were three of the five hospital
nurses Mother Emma Langston took to Balaclava in January 1855. Nightingale
originally thought Disney would be one of her better nurses, probably because she
was a hospital nurse, although that is not recorded. However, Disney was a heavy
drinker, and exhibited what Margaret Wear considered 'violent and unruly conduct'
towards her. Selena Bracebridge considered her 'a most dangerous woman'.[4] Mrs
Jane Gibson, an experienced surgical nurse from St Thomas', was sent to nurse
an officer in his own hut. Her colleagues found her a few hours later, lying on

---

[3]   FNM/LMA/H1/ST/NC8/1, p. 26; WI/Ms/8995/69 and 78; BL 43397, fol. 87.
[4]   WI/Ms/8995/78; FNM/LMA/H1/ST/NC8/1, p. 11.

the floor in a drunken coma.[5] Mrs Whitehead was yet another St Thomas' nurse who came highly recommended. She was a most valuable nurse, who was not dismissed, but had to be invalided home because she broke her leg when drunk.[6]

It is striking how many of the nurses got into trouble at the Balaclava General Hospital under the superintendence of first Langston and then Wear, supporting Nightingale's view of their lack of managerial capacity. Even Mrs Grundy, who was a most efficient nurse, with seven years' experience at the Middlesex, and who was not dismissed, got quite out of hand in Balaclava, although under Nightingale's supervision she did very well. Grundy went home to England in November 1855 because she had received bad news about her children. Nightingale parted with her with great regret.[7] Mrs Gailey was known to Nightingale's family, for Nightingale's mother was helping her son. Nightingale dismissed her because she went out without leave in bad company, presumably drinking.[8]

Of all the nurses who were discharged for major drinking problems, perhaps the most surprising was Mrs Mary Clarke, the matron of the Barrack Hospital. She had been matron of a workhouse in Sheffield, and was Nightingale's matron at Harley Street.[9] Not one of the nurses in Scutari had a kind word for her. She and Mother Mary Clare Moore were in charge of the extra diet kitchen. Sister Sarah Anne Terrot preferred to get the rations for her patients from Moore because she was always patient and helpful, while Clarke scolded the nurses.[10] The St John's House nurses said she all but starved them, and that Nightingale believed everything that this 'low woman' told her about them.[11] Mother Francis Bridgeman said Clarke was frequently very rude,[12] while even the far more generous Mother Mary Clare Moore wrote that Clarke measured out the food to the Sisters in 'scanty quantities' and used the most abusive language to them.[13] Nightingale defended Clarke, saying that although somewhat brusque, she set 'an example of incessant labour'.[14] Nightingale always admired a hard worker, and Clarke had been 'an army in itself' as matron at Harley Street.[15] However, when in April 1855 it was discovered that Clarke was a heavy drinker and encouraged others to get drunk, Nightingale dismissed her. Presumably because of her long service

---

[5]   Davis, *The Autobiography of Elizabeth Davis*, vol. 2, pp. 133–4.

[6]   Ibid., p. 187; FNM/LMA/H1/ST/NC8/1, p. 11.

[7]   FNM/LMA/H1/ST/NC8/1, p. 5; WI/Mss/8995/5, 65 and 78.

[8]   WI/Ms/8995/10, 13 and 78.

[9]   M. Bostridge, *Florence Nightingale: The Making of an Icon* (New York, 2008), p. 185.

[10]   Terrot, *Reminiscences of Scutari Hospitals*, pp. 44–5, 101–2.

[11]   LMA/H01/ST/NC3/SU13, 15, 16.

[12]   Bridgeman, 'An Account', p. 138.

[13]   BA/Annals, 1855, pp. 252–3.

[14]   LMA/H1/ST/NC3/SU18.

[15]   WI/Ms/8994/87.

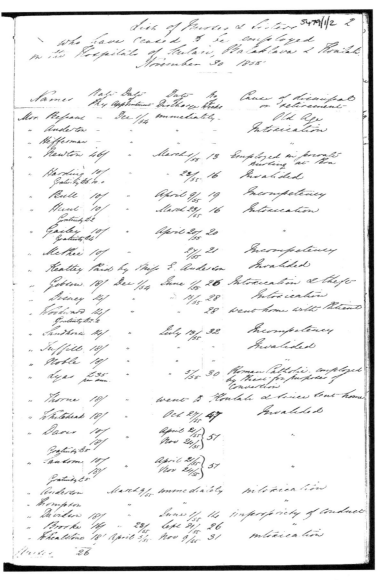

Figure 6.2     Page from Nightingale's list of nurses who returned to England,
1854–55. Altogether 64 nurses returned to England during the
first year of the war, some because they were dismissed, and some
because they were too ill to work. Intoxication and incompetence
were the two commonest reasons for dismissal.

*Source*: Wellcome Library, London, by kind permission.

Nightingale gave the cause of her leaving as illness rather than dismissal, and gave her a gratuity of £8.[16]

Other nurses were dismissed for suspected proselytizing, inexperience and the standard failure to follow doctors' orders. Mrs Lyas claimed she was the daughter of a French officer who was killed at Waterloo, and said she had trained in both English and French hospitals. Nightingale dismissed her because she thought one of the Catholic priests was employing her to help him convert nurses.[17] Nightingale dismissed four of the six St John's House nurses in January 1855. Three were quite inexperienced – one had only just completed her three months' probation ten days before leaving for Scutari[18] – but Mother Mary Clare Moore commented: 'They were of a more respectable class than the hospital nurses'.[19] Nightingale, however, preferred the less respectable nurses who were more clinically experienced, and she would not tolerate nurses who gave the men food and drink without a doctor's order, as these four nurses did.[20]

## Disorderliness and Levity of Conduct

All the ladies were anxious to prevent the nurses from socially disgracing the new venture of female nurses in military hospitals, and hence emphasized propriety, a middle-class standard which many did not meet. Maria Parkes discharged Marion Hepburn for 'disorderly conduct' and an indifferent character.[21] Mrs Susannah Faulkner came from a group originally organized by Dr Acland in Oxford during the cholera epidemic. After the cholera abated, this group, under the direction of philanthropist Felicia Skene, continued to do district nursing. Nightingale considered Skene's nurses less skilled than the hospital nurses, for she paid them 16s. a week rather than the 18s. she gave her best hospital nurses. Faulkner was sent home for disobedience; she walked out with soldiers and conducted herself 'in a disreputable manner'.[22] Mrs Davidson was an experienced head nurse from the famous Dr Simpson's ward at the Edinburgh Royal Infirmary. She was trustworthy and highly respectable, but Nightingale dismissed her for what Selena Bracebridge described as disobedience to orders and 'lightness of conduct'.[23]

What was disobedience to orders and lightness of conduct in a trustworthy and respectable woman? Could it have been a lack of deference, as Anne Summers

[16]   WI/Mss/8995/11 and 78.
[17]   WI/Ms/8995/78; FNM/LMA/H1/ST/NC8/1, p. 9.
[18]   LMA/H01/ST/SJ/A20/2, 30 January 1854; LMA/H01/ST/SJ/A20/3, 14 June 1854; LMA/H01/ST/SJ/C1/1, pp. 147, 149.
[19]   BA/Annals/1854, p. 226.
[20]   LMA/H01/ST/NC3/SU14.
[21]   BL 43402, fol. 2.
[22]   FNM/LMA/H1/ST/NC8/1, p. 21.
[23]   WI/Ms/8995/78; FNM/LMA/H1/ST/NC8/1, pp. 17–18.

implied?[24] This seems unlikely, for while Margaret Wear and Selena Bracebridge were distressed by the lack of deference of some nurses, Nightingale put up with a very great deal if the nurses were competent, as for example in the case of Martha Wheatstone. It was probably not flirting, for Nightingale kept on Ruth Dawson, who constantly flirted with the officers,[25] as well as Mrs McPherson, who although 'perfectly sober, honest, respectable but habitually indolent, was given to flirting although ancient'.[26] In Nightingale's opinion, Dawson's impropriety of manner made her unfit to be an officer's nurse, and a very improper person to be about men at all. Nightingale sensed that she had somehow fallen from a higher social position and felt a deep sense of injury. Her attitude towards women was disrespectful and provoking, and Nightingale thought she was probably trying to marry an officer. Nevertheless, even though she had favourites among her patients, Nightingale considered Dawson one of the best nurses she had ever met, in part because she always carried out medical orders faithfully. For this reason, and also because discipline had been laxer at the Palace Hospital where she was first posted and where the nurses were often treated as companions to the officers, Nightingale kept her until the very last. Nightingale sent the nurses home after the war in several parties, sending the least efficient home first, and the best last.[27]

Perhaps Mrs Mary Ann Clark and Mrs Ann Taunton, whom Nightingale considered the two most troublesome nurses at Scutari, are examples of levity of conduct, or indeed, Mrs Willoughby Moore, who went boating with the officers. This was not quiet, modest, and sober conduct indicating total commitment to the nursing which Nightingale demanded. Clark was kind and industrious, and sent half of her 16s. a week home to her family, but Nightingale thought her manner unsuitable for a military hospital and was always suspicious of her. Taunton was a St Bartholomew's nurse who was perfectly sober and respectable, a good active nurse, trustworthy and truthful, but not as devoted to the work as Nightingale felt nurses should be. Taunton was much given to thoughts of marriage, which Nightingale found 'inconvenient' in a hospital nurse in the field. She made love to an orderly, who turned out to be a married man, so Nightingale placed her in a set of wards with a religious Sister. Taunton rebelled, hoping that Nightingale would remove the Sister, but instead Nightingale removed Taunton, which vexed her so much that she became ill. Although Nightingale seriously considered sending her back to England sooner, she kept her to the very end because of her extensive nursing knowledge.[28]

One famous nurse who came to Balaclava, Mary Seacole, often called the black Florence Nightingale, may be the best illustration of what the ladies considered light conduct. She is also an example of an independent entrepreneurial nurse,

[24]   Summers, *Angels and Citizens*, pp. 21–2.
[25]   BL 43397, fols 133–4.
[26]   BL 43402, fol. 11.
[27]   Ibid., fols 4–6; BL 43397, fols 133–4.
[28]   WI/Ms/8995/26; FNM/LMA/H1/ST/NC8/1, p. 26.

although she preferred to call herself a 'doctress'. When she applied to the ladies who recruited the nurses in London, they rejected her. She then went to the Crimea in partnership with a businessman and established what she called the British Hotel, a store with every type of article, a mess table and comfortable quarters for sick and convalescent officers who paid for their care. Lady Alicia Blackwood, who ran a hospital and a store for the soldiers' wives, thought Seacole's prices quite high, in fact slightly usurious. On the other hand, Seacole gave freely to those who could not pay. She frequently visited the battlefields, something Nightingale's nurses were not allowed to do, giving medical aid and refreshments to soldiers as well as officers. She served hot tea almost every day to the wounded as they were being loaded on to the transports for Scutari. However, she also provided 'good cheer' and cooling drinks for the horse races, dog hunts, cricket matches and dinner parties which became so popular in May 1855.[29]

Seacole was certainly trustworthy, and now commands enormous respect in the current sense of the word, but her conduct was not 'sober' in the sense of the quiet, serious, behaviour which Nightingale expected and which had been demanded of the Kaiserswerth deaconesses. Nightingale thought the British Hotel, though not a brothel, something very close to it. She said Seacole was very kind to both men and officers, but was also the cause of much drunkenness and improper conduct – in short, a corrupting influence. 'I had the greatest difficulty in repelling Mrs Seacole's advances,' she wrote later, 'and in preventing association between her and my nurses.'[30] It is worthwhile pointing out that this independent, entrepreneurial nurse, so well loved by the soldiers, had no impact on the development of nursing.

Gross misconduct, usually a euphemism for sexual relations, was a great worry not only among the lady nurses, but among the doctors. 'I am afraid', George Lawson wrote when he heard that female nurses were coming to Balaclava:

> that with all Miss Nightingale's care and looking after her charges, she will not be able to put a stop to a number of little amours and intrigues which are sure to be carried on amongst a lot of comparatively healthy men who have nothing but an injury, which in many cases may be slight.[31]

Mrs Mary Ann Brown was discharged for gross misconduct and drunkenness. Mrs Mary Young, a surgical nurse from Bart's was dismissed on suspicion of 'very gross misconduct'. Mrs Sarah Jones, another of Miss Skene's district nurses, left in disgrace. Nightingale called her a reckless liar who had been meeting

---

[29]    Lady A. Blackwood, *A Narrative of Personal Experience and Impressions during a Residence on the Bosphorus during the Crimean War* (London, 1881), pp. 262–3; Mary Seacole, *The Wonderful Adventures of Mrs Seacole* (London, 1857), pp. 127–8, 135–6, 189–90; Bonham-Carter, *Surgeon in the Crimea*, pp. 156–7, 192 n. 4.

[30]    WI/Ms/9004/60.

[31]    Bonham-Carter, *Surgeon in the Crimea*, p. 163.

clandestinely with a lover.[32] The only domiciliary nurse recruited was Mary Grey, a widow who had been doing private nursing for seven years. She was discharged for intoxication and impropriety of conduct.[33]

A number of the nurses were inefficient, but not so bad as to merit dismissal. Mrs Mary Ann Davis was the widow of a coal merchant; she was sober, honest and respectable, but indolent. Mrs Michael was a respectable woman, but a selfish and indifferent nurse. Mrs Crockitt was a good nurse, but used bad language, which Victorians considered an addiction as bad as drinking.[34]

A much larger number of the working-class women were good nurses, but had some major problem, of which drinking, as already noted, was the most common. Elizabeth Hawkins is an excellent example. She was a widow who came highly recommended from Guy's Hospital, where she had been a night nurse for two months. She lived in Nightingale's neighbourhood, and sent money home for her nephew via Nightingale's family. She may have volunteered after the first party left, and was advised to get hospital experience as Jane Shaw Stewart did. Hawkins was active, clean, very industrious, strictly honest and kind, but drank – a weakness which she struggled hard to overcome.[35] 'Hawkins has been sober two whole days,' Nightingale wrote the Bracebridges in August 1855:

> the results of my having locked up the Brandy in our sitting-room in the closet in the kitchen & keeping the key. But she never wants *now* to clean the Sitting room nor even offers to do anything tho' she protested the very day after you went away she was always ready to clean.[36]

Nightingale was very fond of her, and would keep her until the very last.[37]

Mrs Davey and Mrs Parker both had drinking problems. Nevertheless, because they were such good nurses, Nightingale kept them on for the duration of the war. She became as fond of Davey as she was of Hawkins. Davey was a good nurse, but deteriorated in terms of sobriety and propriety during the war. She was most anxious to do her duty, worked hard and well, was good-hearted, clever, had a tender conscience, and like Hawkins, struggled hard and generally with success against her fondness for drink. Mrs Parker was a kind-hearted, clever nurse who, like Davey, never denied her follies, but, Nightingale said, was perfectly incapable of construing the words propriety and sobriety.[38] Mrs Tandy, who also had a weakness for drink, was another one of Nightingale's best nurses. She had been a

[32]   FNM/LMA/H1/ST/NC8/1, pp. 20–21; BL 43402, fols 4, 7.

[33]   FNM/LMA/H1/ST/NC8/1, p. 28.

[34]   Ibid., pp. 24, 16, 15; Taylor, *Eastern Hospitals and English Nurses*, 1st edn, vol. 1, pp. 235–6.

[35]   WI/Ms/8995/14 and 21; BL 43402, fols 3, 6.

[36]   WI/Ms/8995/26.

[37]   BL 43402, fols 3, 6.

[38]   Ibid., fols 5, 6, 13.

nurse at Bart's for five years. She was in the last group of nurses to be sent home, for she was 'one of the cleverest, handiest and most useful women' Nightingale had ever met, an excellent cook, a good nurse and a good servant.[39]

It has been suggested that the ladies were not prepared to meet the working-class women on their own terms, but rather they assumed a mistress–servant relationship.[40] This was true of Selena Bracebridge and Margaret Wear, but nurses such as Davey, Parker, Tandy and Dawson demonstrate that the lady superintendents were more interested in nursing skill and knowledge than in obedient, deferential nurses. They were quite willing to keep on nurses who drank or were not respectful as long as they were able to do good nursing work.

## The Importance of Clinical Experience

Nearly all the nurses whom the lady superintendents characterized as excellent had hospital experience. Mrs Brownlow was an exception. Nightingale found her in the maternity hospital which Lady Alicia Blackwood started in the basement of the Barrack Hospital, and originally hired her because she had a newborn baby. She lived in Nightingale's house and did the laundry, cooked extra diets, and looked after the sick nurses whom Nightingale usually boarded in her home. Brownlow was always sober, respectable, honest and industrious.[41] Nor is any previous nursing experience mentioned for Mrs Bull, the widow of a major in the militia whom Selena Bracebridge characterized as 'perfectly useless'. Sister Sarah Anne Terrot thought otherwise. She said Bull mothered the men with tender and watchful care, petting and coaxing them with spoonfuls of jelly and beef tea. Bull was also able to check the neglect of the 'wild, rough boys' who acted as orderlies.[42]

Three of the best nurses were Elizabeth Fry nurses, while two came from St John's House. The two St John's House nurses were Elizabeth Woodward and Elizabeth Drake. Nightingale characterized Woodward as 'a very superior woman. With strong religious principle – & so trustworthy that it appears hardly respectful to her to enumerate her good qualities', but her delicate health prevented her from doing heavy work. Nightingale used her largely as a housekeeper and supervisor.[43]

Drake's history gives us a poignant insight into one kind of working-class nurse at mid-century. Drake, whom Nightingale considered 'invaluable, kind, careful,

[39]   FNM/LMA/H1/ST/NC8/1, p. 18; BL 43402, fol. 24.

[40]   Summers, 'Ministering Angels', pp. 142, 144–5; Summers, 'Pride and Prejudice: Ladies and Nurses in the Crimean War', *History Workshop*, 16 (1983): pp. 33–56.

[41]   FNM/LMA/H01/ST/NC8/1, p. 32; BL 43402, fol. 12.

[42]   FNM/LMA/H01/ST/NC8/1, p. 10; Terrot, *Reminiscences of Scutari Hospitals*, pp. 101–2.

[43]   FNM/LMA/H01/ST/NC8/1, p. 7; BL 43402, fol. 13; Bonham-Carter, *Surgeon in the Crimea*, pp. 175, pp. 193–4 n. 9.

modest',[44] entered St John's House as a probationer in January 1854, and was admitted as a nurse three months later. She then did mostly domiciliary nursing. Her patients all commented on her gentle and respectful manner, unwearying good temper and 'exceedingly civil, obliging, quiet, well conducted' behaviour.[45] When in August 1855 she died of fever in Balaclava, Nightingale said she had never thought Drake would be long-lived – she was not attached to life, for she had suffered very much in it.[46]

Nearly all of the remaining first-class nurses had extensive hospital experience, three in lunatic asylums. Mrs Eliza Sullivan had been a nurse for five and a half years at the Colney Hatch Lunatic Asylum. She was an excellent nurse, a most trustworthy woman, perfectly sober, kind and attentive, zealous and honest. She was later promoted to the linen stores, a job normally reserved for the ladies, where she proved very efficient.[47] Janet Duncan and Sarah Grove came from the Edinburgh Lunatic Asylum. They were sober, honest, respectable and kind, and Duncan was one of the best medical nurses.[48]

Elizabeth Smith had six or seven years' experience at St Thomas'. She was a very steady, deserving woman.[49] Mrs Barker, although self-willed, was perfectly sober, respectable, hard-working, trustworthy and honest, and had strong religious principles. She was a good nurse: cooking and housekeeping were her forte. She could cook single-handed all the extra diets for one hospital.[50] Mrs Robbins had four and a half years' experience in the Female Accident Ward at the Birmingham Queen's Hospital. She was sober, respectable, a kind and excellent nurse, and a good and active cook for hospital extras.[51] Mrs Elizabeth Logan came from Edinburgh, and was sober, respectable, a kind and excellent surgical nurse, very clever at her business, industrious, and thoroughly trustworthy. She was also a good washerwoman, and very clean. Nightingale later described her as 'the most respectable and sober, efficient, kind & good of all my nurses – the one I most hope not to lose sight of – the one I have the deepest regard for'.[52]

Mrs Tuffill had worked at King's College Hospital for two years, and was a clever, useful woman. Even Selena Bracebridge was impressed by her, describing her as an excellent nurse who behaved extremely well. Her motive for going to Scutari was to nurse her second husband, who was a soldier. Nightingale assigned her to him as his private nurse when he was dying, and later commented acerbically that she was 'wild with despair' when he died and anxious to go home,

44    FNM/LMA/H1/ST/NC3/SU14.
45    LMA/H01/ST/SJ/A20/2, 30 January, 1 May 1854; LMA/H01/ST/SJ/C3/1, p. 123.
46    FNM/LMA/H1/ST/NC3/SU35.
47    WI/Ms/8996/69; FNM/LMA/H1/ST/NC8/1, p. 26.
48    FNM/LMA/H1/ST/NC8/1, pp. 29, 30.
49    Ibid., p. 5.
50    BL 43402, fol. 11; FNM/H1/ST/NC8/1, p. 17.
51    FNM/H1/ST/NC8/1, p. 10; WI/Mss/8995/21; BL 43402, fol. 24.
52    LMA/H01/ST/NC8/1, p. 26; BL 42403, fol. 24; BL 43397, fol. 129.

but not before she became engaged to a third husband. In the event, she stayed until she was invalided home when her health collapsed due to overwork caring for her patients.[53] Mrs Holmes had three years' experience at the London Hospital, and was most correct in her conduct and an indefatigable, judicious and excellent nurse whose sobriety was unquestionable. The doctors liked her very much, but she became engaged to a soldier and returned home to be married.[54]

Mrs Mary Ann Noble was an experienced nurse from the Westminster Hospital. She went to Balaclava in January 1855. She and Jane Shaw Stewart had originally planned to work on the ships which transported the wounded to Scutari, but they decided they were needed even more in the Crimean hospitals. Nightingale considered Noble one of the best, kindest, most proper, most skilful surgical nurses in the two hospitals at Balaclava. She recommended an extra year's salary for her when she was invalided home.[55]

Susan Cator was another first-class nurse. She had had long experience at the London Hospital, first as an assistant nurse for 11 years starting when she was about 22, and then as a head nurse for eight years. Nightingale had a real affection for her because she was an excellent nurse, indefatigable with her patients, a sensible woman, and perfect in propriety and sobriety. After the war, she was one of the nurses whom Nightingale had her mother entertain at the family home, and she found her a job as a sister at St Thomas'.[56] Long experience as a sister in a teaching hospital, however, was not necessarily an indication of an expert nurse. Mrs Rogers, who was appointed sub-matron at the Renkioi Hospital, had been a sister at Guy's for nineteen years. She had excellent references, but proved quite incompetent as a sub-matron.[57]

Of all the hospital nurses, Nightingale rated Eliza Roberts the best. Thirty-six years after the war, Roberts stood out in her mind as a 'splendid nurse and excellent woman'. Roberts started at St Thomas' as an assistant nurse on men's surgery in 1829. Eleven years later she became sister of George Ward, a men's surgical and accident ward. In 1853, after 24 years at St Thomas' and not yet 50 years old, she retired due to failing health. Nightingale recognized her exceptional competence immediately, saying only ten days after arriving in Scutari that Roberts was worth her weight in gold. She became Nightingale's head nurse – Dr Peter Pincoffs, a civilian doctor, called her Nightingale's 'clever aide-de-camp'. Nightingale believed she could have been a first-rate surgeon and physician, and accordingly paid her £65 a year,[58] more than she paid any other nurse.

---

53   FNM/H1/ST/NC8/1, p. 10; BL 47717, fol. 44.

54   FNM/H1/ST/NC8/1, p. 18; BL 43402, fols 5, 6.

55   Davis, *The Autobiography of Elizabeth Davis*, vol. 2, p. 141; BL 43396, fol. 35.

56   LH/F11/4, p. 38; LMA/H1/ST/C2, no pagination; FNM/H1/ST/NC8/1, p. 31; BL 43402, fol. 16; LMA/H1/ST/NC1/V48/56.

57   FNM/H1/ST/NC8/1, p. 17.

58   BL 47724, fol. 195; LMA/H1/ST/C2/1; LMA/H1/ST/D7/21, p. 150; Nightingale to William Bowman, 14 November 1854, Bowman Private Collection; P. Pincoffs,

Richard Whitfield, the apothecary and senior resident medical officer at St Thomas', also thought Roberts the best nurse he had ever known,[59] while the army surgeons were particularly impressed by her. Nightingale attributed her nursing expertise to her many years of experience at St Thomas'. She had skills which few other nurses had in the 1850s, because by then the dressers had taken over so much of what the surgical sisters formerly did. 'Her total superiority to all the vices of a Hospital Nurse, her faithfulness to the work, her disinterested love of duty & vigilant care of her Patients, her power of work equal to that of *ten* nurses,' Nightingale wrote, 'have made her one of the most important persons of the expedition.'[60]

Roberts became the mainstay of Nightingale's working-class staff. Yet her crude manners made her a difficult employee. She was barely literate, used bad language and talked incessantly. She became angry with people for tiring Nightingale with talk, and yet she herself repeated disturbing stories over and over again. She quarrelled constantly and was proud of it, calling herself 'pepper'. At one point Nightingale said that if Roberts were to leave, she herself would have to resign and go home. Roberts was well aware of Nightingale's dependence on her, and if Nightingale reprimanded her for any of her failings, she would simply threaten to resign and return to England.[61] Like most of the other lady superintendents, Nightingale had more respect for professional expertise than for social etiquette, and was fully prepared to put up with Roberts's uncouthness in exchange for her excellent nursing skills.

An analysis of the way the working-class nurses functioned indicates that the strict discipline which the lady superintendents enforced was quite necessary when dealing with those women who had real nursing expertise but whose lack of self-restraint vitiated their competencies. Nor was it possible to make the most of these women's nursing abilities without first inculcating what the Victorians called moral values – in this case the need for consistency, self-control, working together as a team and implementing doctors' orders. The character elevation on which Anne Ward Morton spent so much energy, and the discipline and sobriety which the ladies tried to encourage, were essential for the promotion of nursing proficiency.

None of the Crimean War nurses had the cruel streak which Dickens's fictional hospital nurse Betsy Prigg had, but cruelty, or 'harsh treatment of the patients', was a not infrequent occurrence, as we have seen, in the London hospitals. It is important to remember that the Crimean War hospital nurses were all hand-picked from a much larger pool of applicants, and came with high recommendations from

*Experiences of a Civilian in Eastern Military Hospitals* (London, 1857), p.78; WI/Ms/7204 Part 2/1 and 8995/78.

[59]   BL 47742, fols 65–6.

[60]   BL 43402, fol. 23 (original emphasis).

[61]   LMA/H1/ST/NC5/3/15; WI/Ms/7204 Part 2//1; BL 47715, fol. 23; O'Malley, *Florence Nightingale*, pp. 344, 352.

doctors and/or the matrons and chaplains of their hospitals. There were certainly some ideal nurses among the war nurses, all the more to be admired for maintaining their integrity amidst such difficult circumstances, but it is worth noting that Eliza Roberts, whom Nightingale said had 'total superiority to all the vices of a hospital nurse', was not free from the wrangling which was so distressing to hospital governors, and the bad language which the ladies so deprecated.

## Military Nursing Work in the 1850s

What were the diseases with which the Crimean War nurses had to deal? Dysentery, chest complaints, frostbite, fever and scurvy were the commonest problems in the first winter, and then came the wounds, which, as opposed to soldiers in the field hospitals, accounted for only a small number of the patients in the base hospitals.[62] Sister Sarah Anne Terrot said that although some of her first patients lingered for a long time, she could not remember one who ultimately survived. While the hospitals were gradually improving in December, January and February, the patients arrived in progressively worse condition. They came devoured by lice, in indescribable states of filth and with death written on their faces. The bearers carried them from ward to ward, searching for a place to lay them down, usually one just emptied by a corpse. The orderlies tried to turn them away. 'We don't want any more of his sort here, we have more already than we can look to,' they would say.[63]

Because there was no nursing care for the men on the transports, many had horrific bedsores covering their neck, back and hips – sores from which they eventually died. Timothy Gowing, a sergeant in the Royal Fusiliers, received bayonet wounds in both thighs at the battle of Inkerman. He was more fortunate than many in being taken to the regimental hospital, where his wounds were dressed and bandaged. He was then shipped to Scutari on an old steamer. There were not enough doctors on board to look after 50 men, much less up to 400, and although they worked like horses, they could not keep up. Gowing found the sight of so many men dying heart-rending. 'Many of our poor fellows had not had the slightest thing done for them since they were wounded on that bloody field,' he wrote, 'and were now left to die in agony and oh! horror of horrors, their poor mangled bodies were infested with vermin.' Men were shrieking with pain, some lying in a state of putrefaction, others dying, and still others being carried up on

---

[62]    Soldiers with medical conditions always vastly outnumbered the wounded, and the wounded, of course, often suffered from medical problems as well. J. Shepherd, *The Crimean Doctors: A History of the British Medical Services in the Crimean War* (2 vols, Liverpool, 1991), vol. 1, pp. 194–200; ibid., vol. 2, pp. 341–8, 518.

[63]    Terrot, *Reminiscences of Scutari Hospitals*, pp. 27, 37.

deck to be buried at sea. After four or five days, when the steamer reached Scutari, the hospital was full and it had to go on to Malta.[64]

Martha Nicol, one of the Smyrna nurses, reported that fever, often the worst kind of spotted typhus, at one point was killing ten men a day. As the winter progressed, a significant number of patients suffered from rheumatism, but the nurses considered frostbite the worst affliction. 'To my dying day I can never forget the dreadful frostbite' at Scutari and Koulali, the very experienced Sister Mary Aloysius Doyle wrote. No matter what care they got, the men were so prostrate that they could not survive. Their flesh and clothes were frozen together in one piece, their boots having to be cut off, leaving many pieces of flesh in the boots and the sinews and bones of their feet exposed. You could not recognize their toes as such, she said, and frostbite was far more painful than their wounds.[65]

The nurses' work was perhaps more appalling, but their hours were better than in the English hospitals. The schedule at the Scutari General Hospital was typical. Around 8.30 a.m. the nurses left the Barrack Hospital where they slept and walked the half mile to the General Hospital. Until the dressers arrived at the end of December, the nurses did all the dressings. In January, with the larger number of nurses plus the dressers, a new arrangement was made whereby ladies and Sisters generally no longer gave individual patient care, but had had two working-class nurses working under their direction. The nurses returned to the Barrack Hospital at 1 p.m. for lunch, going back at 2 p.m. until 5 p.m. The afternoon work was lighter – feeding some of the weaker patients, reading to some, and more often, writing letters for others.[66]

It was the orderlies' duty to clean the wards and do all the heavier part of the nursing: bringing up the food from the kitchen, lifting the men, making their beds, which they often failed to do, and washing the patients who could not wash themselves, but again they often did not. Terrot preferred to bathe the men herself rather than insist that an unwilling orderly do it. The orderlies generally left the patients' diets by their beds, sometimes out of their reach and out of their sight. They did not feed any patients except those few who had both arms disabled. Every third night, the orderlies were supposed to sit up with their patients, but after an hour or so, they usually lay down and went to sleep. When the orderly officer made his rounds every night to see that all was well, the moment he raised the latch of the door, the orderlies would shout out, 'All right, your honour.' Many a time, Sister Mary Aloysius Doyle said to herself, 'All, all wrong,' but she could not blame the officer for not coming into the wards because they were 'so filled with pestilence, the air so dreadful that to breathe it might cost him his life'. One

---

[64]   T. Gowing, *A Soldier's Experience or A Voice from the Ranks* (Nottingham, 1886), pp. 71–2, 86–7.

[65]   M. Nicol, *Ismeer or Smyrna and its British Hospital in 1855* (London, 1856), pp. 33–5; Taylor, *Eastern Hospitals and English Nurses*, 3rd edn, pp. 156–7; Doyle, 'Memories of the Crimea', pp. 22–3.

[66]   Terrot, *Reminiscences of Scutari Hospitals*, pp. 71–2, 102.

night, the ladies at Koulali finally managed to awaken an orderly to ask what time they should take off a blister. He knew nothing about the blister or the medicines for the men. After that, the ladies relieved the orderlies of night duty.[67]

The orderlies' job was very depressing and demoralizing for young men who, unlike their French counterparts, had had no training in nursing. They were confined 24 hours a day to what was believed to be the highly infectious air of the wards, and had to look after the dying and carry out the dead. They did not try to learn their business, and did not carry out doctors' orders if they could get away with it. In the wards where there were no nurses, the patients were much neglected. One major part of the nursing care, therefore, was encouraging the orderlies to be more attentive to their patients – a duty at which Sisters Mary Aloysius Doyle, Anne Thom and Sarah Anne Terrot excelled.[68] One can understand why Nightingale's ambition immediately after the war was to establish herself in a military hospital where she could train the orderlies.[69]

The nurses' working day was normally much shorter than in the London hospitals, although when they were inundated with a new shipload of sick and wounded, they had to work very long hours. If they worked well with their orderlies, the nurses' duties, with no cleaning, heavy lifting, bedmaking, bathing or carrying food from the kitchen to the wards, were very much lighter than in the teaching hospitals at home. Many Crimean War nurses would have difficulty getting jobs after the war, for some hospital matrons feared they had become too accustomed to easy work.[70]

What did nursing care specifically consist of in the 1850s? In some ways, it is difficult to tell because it was considered indecorous to write about many parts of nursing care. Nutrient enemas, theoretically given by the orderlies, were undoubtedly a large part of it, but they are nowhere mentioned in the nurses' writings. For example, when surgeon George Lawson fell desperately ill with Crimean fever, his doctor saved his life by '*pouring* brandy down his throat' and giving him strong beef tea enemas.[71]

F.B. Smith and Anne Summers emphasized the domestic aspect of Crimean War nursing,[72] and with good reason, as we have seen, because the nurses were always responsible for the laundry, a large part of the cooking, and in the army hospitals, seeing that the orderlies did their jobs. There was, however, much more to their work than providing the laundry, cooking and 'comforts' which ladies like

[67]    Ibid., p. 72, 39, 103; Taylor, *Eastern Hospitals and English Nurses*, 1st edn, vol. 1, pp. 279–80. See also BL 43393, fols 78–80; Doyle, 'Memories of the Crimea', p. 22.

[68]    Terrot, *Reminiscences of Scutari Hospitals*, pp. 38–9, 64, 68–9; Taylor, *Eastern Hospitals and English Nurses*, 1st edn, vol. 1, pp. 203, 224–46.

[69]    BL 43397, fol. 240.

[70]    See, for example, LMA/H01/ST/NC1/V10/56, V59/56, V40/56, V42/56.

[71]    Bonham-Carter, *Surgeon in the Crimea*, p. 176 (original emphasis).

[72]    F.B. Smith, *Florence Nightingale: Reputation and Power* (Beckenham, Kent, 1982), pp. 43–4; Summers, *Angels and Citizens*, pp. 48–51.

Wear enjoyed giving. Everything was in short supply in that first terrible winter, but the situation was rectified in a remarkably short time. The government began spending a huge amount of money on its military machine, so that the Crimean forces were well supplied by the following summer,[73] and the nurses no longer lacked equipment or provisions.

If the ladies did not give full accounts of all the nursing treatments, they nevertheless left descriptions of a great deal of their work. Frostbite was treated with large linseed or oiled poultices, wounds with stupes[74] and poultices, and cholera with chloroform poultices and massage. Ice packs, when an ice ship came in, were used to allay diarrhoea, dysentery and vomiting. Fever patients required incessant watching and large amounts of fluids and stimulants. Even the fomentations were often made with brandy.[75] A patient whose left arm was utterly useless as a result of chronic exposure in the trenches was blistered, leeched and repeatedly cupped.[76] The soldiers also very much appreciated eau de cologne, which the nurses put on a handkerchief and placed on their pillows to counteract the pervasive offensive smells. Turning and positioning immobile patients with cushions was a major duty, theoretically of the orderlies, but which the ladies frequently performed, and it would appear that even after the dressers came, it was the nurses who cared for the numerous bedsores.[77] Massage was another key nursing treatment. Sister Mary Aloysius Doyle reported that in Scutari, the cholera patients died with such dreadful cramps that one might as well have tried to bend a piece of iron as to move their joints. Nevertheless, she and her orderlies massaged them constantly until they died.[78]

Feeding was of the utmost importance, and providing drinks, especially at night, was a major part of nursing care. Before intravenous therapy, all fluids had to be given by mouth or rectum almost continuously. The most common cases – fever, dysentery, diarrhoea and frostbite – particularly needed fluids. At Koulali these patients were constantly watched, with nurses sometimes putting a piece of ice or a spoonful of wine or beef tea in the patient's mouth every five minutes. For these men, nursing care was more important than medical skill. Solacing the patients was another nursing duty, and could consist of singing:

---

[73]  Hoppen, *The Mid-Victorian Generation*, pp. 179–80; Pincoffs, *Experiences of a Civilian*, pp. 30–31, 55–6.

[74]  A wrung-out flannel or piece of cloth, usually hot and usually medicated, synonymous with fomentation.

[75]  Doyle, 'Memories of the Crimea', pp. 20–23; Goodman, *Experiences of an English Sister of Mercy*, pp. 89–90; Taylor, *Eastern Hospitals and English Nurses*, 3rd edn, p. 70. Fomentation was another name for a stupe or soak.

[76]  Cupping was a method of bleeding which consisted of scarifying (making many small cuts) in the skin and applying a heated cup to the wound.

[77]  Goodman, *Experiences of an English Sister of Mercy*, pp. 129–30; Taylor, *Eastern Hospitals and English Nurses*, 3rd edn, pp. 156–7.

[78]  Doyle, 'Memories of the Crimea', pp. 20–21.

when a civilian doctor was dying, the ladies learned he loved music, so one lady sang to him for hours at a time.[79] With their more holistic concept of health, the nurses helped with letter writing, teaching the convalescent soldiers reading, writing and arithmetic, and giving spiritual consolation of an unsectarian nature and comfort to the dying.[80] Finally, perhaps the nurses' most important function was assessing patients and calling the doctors if they found a man in immediate danger.[81]

## Nursing Expertise in the 1850s: Tact, Training and Judgement

What was 'clever nursing', which is how the ladies usually designated nursing expertise? Was it the mothering, petting and coaxing which Mrs Bull did, or the laundry and cooking which took up so much of the nurses' time? The adjectives which the lady superintendents used most often were 'respectable', 'active', 'clean', 'useful', 'industrious', 'honest', 'kind' and 'sober' – all standard components of Victorian respectability. Propriety, an important part of respectability, was essential. Equally important was the ability to implement the doctors' orders, something which the orderlies as well as many of the old-style hospital nurses frequently failed to do. Ruth Dawson had a poor attitude, but was an excellent nurse because she carried out the doctors' orders faithfully. More important to Nightingale than to the other lady superintendents was total dedication to nursing. Jane Shaw Stewart, though half-mad, had the total dedication which Nightingale so admired. Despite her vulgarity, Eliza Roberts's love of duty, among other things, led Nightingale to rate her as the best of all the hospital nurses.

More than clinical knowledge and respectability was expected from the lady nurses and the best working-class nurses whom the ladies usually described as 'clever nurses'. Mother Mary Clare Moore and Sisters Mary Aloysius Doyle and Anne Thom had gifted administrative skills, bringing order out of chaos and training the orderlies, while by contrast Margaret Wear was able only to nurse individuals. Nursing was one part of the religious Sisters' vocation in life; their thoughts did not wander to marriage or flirting as did those of Taunton or the elderly McPherson. Care of the hospital nurses was another important requisite. Miss Tebbutt's 'anxious care of the nurses' morals' was her one redeeming feature, and Nightingale regretted that other lady superintendents did not keep as watchful an eye on the nurses as she herself did – to the point of locking them

---

[79]  Taylor, *Eastern Hospitals and English Nurses*, 1st edn, vol. 1, pp. 105, 108; ibid., vol. 2, pp. 22–3.

[80]  Goodman, *Experiences of an English Sister of Mercy*, pp. 109, 129–30, 132–3, 154–5, 225.

[81]  Terrot, *Reminiscences of Scutari Hospitals*, p. 63; Goodman, *Experiences of an English Sister of Mercy*, p. 168.

in their quarters at night and sleeping with the key under her pillow.[82] This was to prevent them from going out to spirit houses or to meet soldiers. Locking the nurses in at night was a practice which continued in many English hospitals at least into the early 1890s.[83]

Margaret Goodman perhaps best summed up nursing expertise when she wrote that many of the ladies in the Crimean War thought that the only requirements for a good nurse were a strong constitution and kind intentions. However, their nursing experience soon taught them that 'tact, training and judgement are essentially necessary for those who fill the office of a nurse'.[84] 'Tact' in the nineteenth century had a somewhat different meaning from the modern usage. As well as diplomacy and sensitivity in social relations, it meant a keen faculty of perception or discrimination, likened to a sense of touch. Sometimes 'tact' referred to all five senses, as in 'Sight is a very refined tact.'[85] In 1850 the Boston surgeon Henry Bigelow wanted his students to develop 'surgical tact', the ability to look at operations professionally, to perceive the surgical knowledge and skills being implemented, and not simply the blood, gore and shrieking.[86] In 1864, Dr Symonds of the Bristol Royal Infirmary defined 'nursing tact' as 'a compound result of fine perception and accurate observation, and an instinctive *savoir faire,* and a quickness of imagination'. A nurse with tact saved the doctor many visits, and more importantly, Symonds pointed out, her help enabled the doctor to 'select the very best remedies and methods of treatment'.[87] What would later be called observational skills, and in our time, assessment skills, were part of nursing tact. In addition to tact and training, Goodman pointed out that nurses had to have professional judgement. This is what Sister Mary Jones would define in 1866 as 'common sense' when she described the best nurses as having 'manual skill – knowledge & common-sense'.[88]

Professional judgement, which requires both knowledge and experience, was the paramount quality among the best nurses. For example, Sister Bertha Turnbull had good sense and good judgement, while Mother Francis Bridgeman had a good sense and judgement in nursing attained by few. Susan Cator and Sister Ann Thom were described as 'sensible', an adjective the ladies used frequently as a synonym for 'judicious'. The six Bermondsey Sisters for whom Nightingale wrote characters all had good judgement, as did the best working-class nurses such as Mary Ann Noble and Mrs Holmes. Professional judgement was the quality which earlier doctors such as Graves and Southwood Smith

[82]   LMA/NC18/15, fol. 47.
[83]   BL 47737, fol. 11.
[84]   Goodman, *Experiences of an English Sister of Mercy*, p. 132.
[85]   C.T. Onions (ed.), *Oxford Universal Dictionary* (Oxford, 1955), pp. 2,120–21.
[86]   Stanley, *Hospitals and Sisterhoods*, p. 176.
[87]   *Lancet*, 20 February 1864, pp. 212–13.
[88]   BL 47744, fol. 90.

had looked for, and the lack of which Dr Bence Jones of St George's Hospital decried in Jane Medwinter.

Wars have always been a harsh test of the capabilities of individuals, occupations, institutions and societies, as well as opportunities for rapidly increasing competencies. This was as true of the Crimean War as of any other war. Nightingale and the religious Sisters already had administrative and nursing experience which they honed further during the war. Successful lady superintendents who were not experienced nurses were forced to quickly develop administrative systems which could cope with the shortage of supplies and the soldiers' horrific medical problems during that first terrible winter. In most cases, the best nurses' professional judgement had resulted from their hospital experience. This confirmed Nightingale's belief that clinical experience, preferably in a large teaching hospital, was essential to develop nursing expertise.

Nursing reached a crossroad in the 1850s. Hospital doctors and administrators had been pressing for better nursing for more than a generation, but it was not clear what better nursing would consist of. Would it be grounded in clinical experience and devoted to the bodily needs of the patients, leaving the religious aspects to the chaplains, as Nightingale thought? Or should salvation of the soul be the ultimate goal, as Bridgeman and Stanley believed? Would the new nurses be doctors' ancillaries, simply following their orders, or would their role be essentially domestic, the cooking and feeding which the ladies at Koulali considered the most important part of their work?[89]

Three of Nightingale's five best nurses were religious Sisters. Their discipline, humanity and clinical expertise suggested that religious Sisters would be the leaders of the new nursing. However, political restrictions eliminated the Catholic nuns. The Anglican Sisters' competence and their later brilliant success after the war at three of the London teaching hospitals made it seem as if their nursing system would be the system of the future. But religious prejudices and the Sisters' insistence on running their nursing services themselves would be their undoing.

In 1856, no one would have thought that the working-class hospital nurses would have the greatest influence on the new nursing, but in the end, it was they, not the religious Sisters or the highly touted ladies, who would most strongly influence the shape of modern nursing. The hospital nurses were so badly educated that they could not lead the reforms – Mrs Roberts, for example, despite her extraordinary nursing knowledge, could barely read.[90] Many expert working-class nurses had little self-restraint, and in order to function effectively, required highly disciplined working conditions with close supervision. Harsh discipline and close supervision would become a hallmark of the new nursing, which was an unfortunate legacy of the working-class nurses. However, despite the egregious failings of many, they could handle the long hours of hard physical

---

[89]   Taylor, *Eastern Hospitals and English Nurses*, 3rd edn, pp. 193–6.
[90]   WI/Ms/7204/Part 2/1.

work which nursing demanded. More importantly, the best working-class nurses had extensive clinical experience, a specific body of knowledge and the judgement which by mid-century had become essential for an effective nurse. This was their key legacy, a legacy which the Crimean War lady nurses could not bequeath. Many of the expert hospital nurses in the 1850s were still not the 'proper persons' Dr Golding looked for in 1819, and cooking, cleaning and laundering remained a large part of their duties. More important, however, their knowledge and skills were far more sophisticated than those of the best nurses at the London Hospital in 1824.

# Chapter 7
# St John's House and its Mission

It was the Anglican Sisters, and one Anglican sisterhood in particular, St John's House, which devised a method of systematically training both nurses and sisters with the aim of reforming hospital nursing and meeting the teaching hospitals' ever-expanding demand for efficient nurses. By making nursing sisters religious Sisters, St John's House brought both traditional respectability and the zeal of nineteenth-century religious reform to nursing work.

Providing the eminent respectability which Kaiserswerth offered and combining religious discipline and nurture with instruction and clinical nursing experience in a teaching hospital, the Sisters of St John's House spearheaded nursing reform in England. In 1856 they took over the nursing at King's College Hospital, and in 1866 the nursing at Charing Cross Hospital. Using a modified form of the St John's House system, another Anglican sisterhood, the All Saints Sisters of the Poor, took over the nursing at University College Hospital in 1862. In the 1860s and 1870s these three hospitals became the models for improved nursing in the Protestant English-speaking world. However, as religious Sisters, these nurses also attracted the powerful anti-Catholic prejudices and impassioned religious controversy which characterized nineteenth-century English society.

## The Anglican Sisterhoods

The new Anglican sisterhoods were one result of nineteenth-century Anglican renewal. Susan Mumm estimated that more than 90 Anglican sisterhoods involving 10,000 women were founded between 1845, when the first sisterhood, the Park Village community began, and 1900.[1] Historians have generally given the sisterhoods involved in nursing only cursory recognition, while wrongly ascribing many of the Sisters' most basic and far-reaching reforms to Florence Nightingale and her school at St Thomas' Hospital. The notable exception is Judith Moore's *A Zeal for Responsibility*, which is an analysis of the St John's House Sisters' struggle for professional recognition.[2] While St John's House has attracted some interest, few historians have looked at the All Saints Sisters. In a short article written in 1959, Sydney Holloway concluded that these Sisters failed to adapt to modern

---

[1]  S. Mumm, *Stolen Daughters, Virgin Mothers* (Leicester, 1999), p. 3.
[2]  Moore, *A Zeal for Responsibility*.

medical practice and were financially irresponsible.[3] The Sisters' twentieth-century chaplain and historian Peter Mayhew, in a reversal of the usual 'insider' stance, accepted the argument that the Sisters were financially incompetent.[4]

In 2001, Sioban Nelson revolutionized thinking about religious nurses' impact on nursing with the publication of *Say Little, Do Much*. Referring to Catholic nursing Sisters, she wrote that their faith 'in God's will and belief in the miraculous enabled them to achieve far more than any group of individual women could ever have accomplished'; their religious commitment enabled them to turn hardship and adversity into spiritual exercises in obedience and humility.[5] Other authors since have deepened our understanding of the professionalism of the Catholic religious nurses.[6] While Anglican Sisters did not believe in present-day miracles, they had the same sense of religious mission and the same religious discipline which likewise enabled them to accept terrible conditions and persevere in the interests of more effective nursing of the sick poor. Looking at the work of the Anglican Sisters, Nelson concluded that they did 'important work ... furthering the cause of trained nurses'.[7] A closer look at the nursing history of St John's House and the All Saints Sisters supports and extends Nelson's conclusion.

### The Foundation and Aims of St John's House

Deeply rooted religious prejudice faced these sisterhoods in their major battle to establish better nursing. The evangelical revival of the eighteenth and early nineteenth centuries had been a richly constructive force in English society. However, it was also a source of tremendous hostilities, expressed in the denominational warfare which dominated politics in the 1830s and 1840s.[8] These major political battles were echoed by all kinds of struggles at a lesser level, and had a very destructive effect on the development of nursing reform, and especially on the reforms of the Anglican Sisters.

The religious revival also divided the Anglican Church into three loose factions: the Low Church or Evangelical party, the Broad Church and the High Church. The High Church people stressed continuity with the pre-Reformation Church and adopted rituals from that time. Most of the new sisterhoods, including the All Saints Sisters, were High Church. They wore nuns' habits and often secretly took life-long vows of poverty, chastity and obedience although canon law forbade such vows. The Broad

---

[3]    S.W.F. Holloway, 'The All Saints Sisterhood at University College Hospital 1862–99', *Medical History*, 3 (1959): pp. 153–4.

[4]    P. Mayhew, *All Saints: Birth and Growth of a Community* (Oxford, 1987), p. 110.

[5]    Nelson, *Say Little, Do Much*, pp. 1–2.

[6]    See, for example, B.M. Wall, *Unlikely Entrepreneurs: Catholic Sisters and the Hospital Marketplace 1865–1925* (Columbus, OH, 2005); Libster and McNeil, *Enlightened Charity*.

[7]    Nelson, *Say Little, Do Much*, p. 71.

[8]    Chadwick, *The Victorian Church*, vol. 1, pp. 7–158, 232–309, 440–55.

Church party liked to think of the Anglican Church as a national and comprehensive Church, excluding no one. They emphasized the corporate and interdependent nature of society and stressed Church unity; they also saw education and social reform as the keys to achieving the Christian vision.[9] The Evangelicals emphasized personal conversion and were strongly anti-Catholic, objecting strenuously to anything which smacked of Roman Catholicism, and hence the High Church practices of many of the new sisterhoods. All three parties became involved in nursing reform.

It was a Broad Churchman and an eminent physician, Dr Robert Bentley Todd, who first conceived the idea of a training school for nurses. Todd was Professor of Physiology and General Morbid Anatomy at King's College, a centre of Broad Church activity.[10] In 1837 he published a series of articles in the *British Magazine*, an Anglican journal, calling for fundamental reform of medical education. 'There is no such thing as discipline in any of the schools of medicine,' he declared, adding that instruction consisted of lectures to which half the medical students did not bother to listen. Todd emphasized the importance of clinical education, but as was standard in his time, believed that the religious and moral education of the students was equally as important as their scientific and practical training.[11] He therefore proposed a residential collegiate system at King's, similar to that at Oxford and Cambridge, with students assigned to a particular professor or lecturer as a mentor. 'A primary object in professional education', he wrote:

> is to cast the professional character in a proper mould, to lay a sound scientific foundation, and to form habits moral, mental and professional which will fit the possessor to occupy a station of respectability and usefulness, in his particular calling as well as in society at large.[12]

By 1843, Todd had become the first dean of King's College Medical School, introduced major reforms in medical education, and established a residence in the college for a number of medical students.[13]

---

[9]   Ibid., vol. 1, pp. 167–231, 440–55, 544–5; P.T. Marsh, *The Victorian Church in Decline: Archbishop Tait and the Church of England 1868–1882* (London, 1969), pp. 10–12; T.E. Jones, *The Broad Church: A Biography of a Movement* (New York, 2003), pp. 2–5.

[10]   C. Helmstadter, 'Robert Bentley Todd, St. John's House, and the Origins of Modern Nursing', *Bulletin of the History of Medicine*, 67 (1993): pp. 286–7.

[11]   R.B. Todd, 'Education of Medical Students', *British Magazine*, 11 (1837): pp. 337–8, 460; D. Newsome, *Godliness and Good Learning: Four Studies of a Victorian Ideal* (London, 1961), pp. 1–2.

[12]   R.B. Todd, *On the Resources of King's College, London, for Medical Education* (London, 1852); R.B. Todd, 'Education of Medical Students', *British Magazine*, 12 (1837): pp. 98–9, 337–40, citation on p. 340.

[13]   F.J.C. Hearnshaw, *Centenary History of King's College London 1828–1928* (London, 1929), pp. 116–17, 139–42; H.W. Lyle, *King's and Some King's Men* (London, 1935), pp. 40–42.

Todd then turned his attention to the problem of hospital nursing. In 1847 he enlisted the support of a group of prominent Anglicans, headed by Bishop Charles James Blomfield, who was his patient and close friend.[14] All who were conversant with the condition of English hospitals, the *British Magazine* explained in 1848, 'are well aware of the difficulty of obtaining good and efficient nurses'.[15] Todd's solution was to develop a class of nurses who would regard their work as a religious calling.[16]

The training school, which opened in 1849, was officially named the Order of St John the Evangelist, but was better known as St John's House. It was also called the Training Institution for Nurses for Hospitals, Families, and the Sick Poor, serving the same areas as Elizabeth Fry's nursing institution. St John's House was based on the same principles as Todd's reforms of medical education at King's: clinical training in the hospital combined with religious education and a residential home with supervision and support from older, better-educated persons. Unpaid upper-class ladies formed the religious sisterhood, and originally only they were to be sisters in the sense of hospital head nurses. The Sisters trained and paid working-class women to be assistant nurses. The paid working-class women were considered members of St John's House, but were not religious Sisters.[17] In the class-bound society of mid-nineteenth-century England, only ladies could be Sisters.

Hospitals had long been searching for respectable, efficient nurses, but the founders of St John's House made it clear that they required more – nurses had to have nursing expertise. 'A nurse may bear a good character,' they explained:

> she may be regular and orderly in her conduct and of strict integrity; she may keep her wards clean and perform her ordinary duties to the perfect satisfaction of her superiors, but may be a very unsafe person to be left in charge of a critical case.

The reform of nursing could not depend on individual efforts (as the ward system did), the *British Magazine* declared. Rather, if there was to be a steady supply of good nurses, there must be systematic training and discipline in an institution organized for that specific purpose.[18]

As with Todd's medical reforms, the aim was to develop nursing expertise through systematic, professional training. This training would elevate character,

[14]   LMA/H01/ST/SJ/A1/1, 19 November 1847; LMA/H01/ST/SJ/A2/1, 12 February 1860.

[15]   Cited in Stanley, *Hospitals and Sisterhoods*, p. 42.

[16]   CSSJD, 'Public Meeting, 13 July 1848', pp. 13–14, 18–19; Stanley, *Hospitals and Sisterhoods*, pp. 42–3.

[17]   CSSJD, Proposed Rules of the Training Institution 1848.

[18]   Stanley, *Hospitals and Sisterhoods*, pp. 44–6, citation on p. 42.

and in the case of the working-class nurses, improve their social status.[19] The emphasis on character elevation was not restricted to nurses or the working classes, but, as Todd had explained, was considered an essential aspect of professional education. For the ladies who were the Sisters, the goal was to provide a legitimate field of labour, either full-time or part-time.[20] Providing work for ladies was a radical move, but was in keeping with Broad Church principles which fostered education for women.[21]

Most early Victorians identified morality with religion: for them, law and social order was based on Christian teaching. To this generation, religious discipline meant education, good order and professionalism as well as the ethical principles we now associate with the term. Furthermore, the Church of England was the state Church, one of the pillars of government and a primary force in education, law and order.[22] In 1839, Lord John Russell, later a major Prime Minister but then Home Secretary, expressed conventional belief when he emphasized that '*first, religious instruction*' should characterize any education offered to the general populace. Then, in Russell's scheme, came general instruction, moral training and habits of industry. His class believed this kind of education for the masses would stabilize the riotous, disorderly society of his time.[23]

These assumptions were the principal reason why Todd and his board chose a sisterhood as the vehicle for the nurses' training school. A sisterhood reflected these values, and conveyed unassailable respectability on the working-class nurses and made the menial work of nursing an act of charity for ladies. Rather than 'low, disorderly, almost sottish women', as Bence Jones had characterized them, the working-class nurses became what Sister Caroline Lloyd would later call 'churchwomen'.[24] When the founders announced the training school's establishment to the public, they emphasized its similarity to the work of religious orders in Catholic countries and Kaiserswerth in Prussia. They emphasized the backing of the Church, naming the Archbishop of York and six other bishops who were sponsoring the project, and explaining that the institution would be 'under the immediate supervision of a clergyman'.[25]

Another very important reason for making the training institution a sisterhood was that a sisterhood allowed ladies to work full-time without losing their status

[19]   LMA/H01/ST/SJ/A17/1.

[20]   Ibid.

[21]   M. Bryant, *The Unexpected Revolution: A Study in the History of the Education of Women and Girls in the Nineteenth Century* (London, 1979), pp. 70–72.

[22]   Chadwick, *The Victorian Church*, vol. 1, pp. 1–3.

[23]   Cited in Rigg, *National Education*, pp. 289–96 (original emphasis).

[24]   LMA/H01/ST/SJ/A39/20, p. 4.

[25]   *The Times*, 17 February 1848, p. 8. See also LMA/H01/ST/SJ/A1/1, 19 November 1847.

as ladies. Christian philanthropy, as numerous historians have shown,[26] provided ladies with a major escape route from the demands of family and the intricacies of upper-class Victorian social life, but their visiting, teaching and social work were only a part-time escape. By contrast, as religious Sisters, ladies could maintain their social status and undertake full-time philanthropic work. As historians Susan Mumm and Martha Vicinus have emphasized, a large part of the appeal of sisterhoods was that they permitted women to lead independent lives and do constructive work; besides, there was a sense of daring and deep fulfilment in helping to reclaim the lives of the poor,[27] and equally important, sisterhoods offered ladies a comfortable home where they could make their own rules and organize their own lives. 'Joining a convent was one of the few assertions of independence which a Victorian woman could make,' Theodore Hoppen wrote, 'and contemporary Protestant critics who saw convent life as a denial of freedom profoundly misunderstood its character.'[28]

St John's House was a real sisterhood, but it differed from the other new Anglican sisterhoods in many ways. First, nearly all the other sisterhoods were founded by ladies and developed from small groups who helped their rector with his parochial work. These ladies ran their sisterhoods themselves; ultimate authority rested within the sisterhood. By contrast, a group of men formed the St John's House Council, as they called their board. They first designed the sisterhood, and then recruited ladies to it. Ultimate authority was vested in the council, not the Sisters. Secondly, because St John's House was a Broad Church foundation, it was a 'lay sisterhood'. The Sisters took no vows of poverty, chastity and obedience; they did not wear nuns' habits; they were prohibited from bringing a dowry; they did not need to live in the community house; they could be married or single; work a few days a week or just several months of the year.[29] For example, after the Crimean War, Anne Ward Morton worked at King's College Hospital from Monday evening through Thursday evening, going home every weekend.[30]

St John's House was also different in its approach to nursing. Although nearly all the sisterhoods did some nursing as well as social work and teaching, St John's House was the only Anglican sisterhood devoted exclusively to nursing.

---

[26]    See, for example, F.K. Prochaska, *Women and Philanthropy in Nineteenth Century England* (London, 1988) pp. 11–17.

[27]    M. Vicinus, *Independent Women: Work and Community for Single Women 1850–1920* (Chicago, IL, 1985), pp. 48–51; Mumm, *Stolen Daughters, Virgin Mothers*, pp. 3, 13–15. Florence Nightingale's 'Cassandra' remains the ultimate cry of despair of a middle-class Victorian woman facing a purposeless life. See Florence Nightingale, *Cassandra and Other Selections from Suggestions for Thought*, ed Mary Poovey (New York, 1992).

[28]    Hoppen, *The Mid-Victorian Generation*, p. 461.

[29]    CSSJD, Proposed Rules 1848; Public Meeting 13 July 1848, pp. 1–4; J.H. Overton and E. Wordsworth, *Christopher Wordsworth, Bishop of Lincoln, 1807–85* (London, 1888), pp. 124–5.

[30]    BL Add Mss 47744, fols 59–60.

Nursing historians have largely dismissed the sisterhoods' contribution to nursing knowledge, arguing that they had little or no specific clinical skills.[31] This was far from the case. Lady Sisters and working-class nurses trained *together* in teaching hospitals – a radical innovation in the strictly segregated class society of the time. Even more radically, and despite later assumptions by historians, before St John's House took over the nursing at King's College Hospital in 1856, experienced working-class nurses and head nurses taught the lady probationers.[32]

A new division of labour was another innovation of St John's House. When the nurses started their training in the hospitals, the Sisters specified they were to do no cleaning nor scrubbing, not even washing dishes: their duties were exclusively attendance on the sick.[33] Yet another major innovation was the nurses' home. The Sisters and their nurses did not live in the miserable quarters hospitals provided, but in an elegant part of London, first in Fitzroy Square, then in Queen's Square, Westminster (now called Queen Anne's Gate), and finally in Norfolk Street, the Strand. Both lady and working-class probationers went out to their hospitals every day in the morning and returned to their comfortable, respectable home in the evening.[34] Later, when St John's House took over hospital nursing services, the nurses did live in the hospitals, but the sisterhood insisted on much-improved accommodation.

Elizabeth Fry's nurses and St John's House shared a number of characteristics. Both societies demanded respectability and provided their nurses with some hospital training. While both made major fundraising efforts, both relied primarily on the fees from nursing in private families for their main source of income. Both had comfortable nurses' homes, and both were modelled in part on Protestant sisterhoods on the Continent such as Kaiserswerth, as well as on the Catholic Sisters of Charity.[35]

Despite these similarities, St John's House was a religious sisterhood, and therefore a very different kind of organization. Todd believed Elizabeth Fry's institution was 'an excellent and useful society', but would have been more useful if it had been a religious organization.[36] St John's House was also different, in that it drew heavily on the model of the new, largely Anglican, training schools for schoolteachers. In the late 1830s and 1840s the Anglicans became leaders in training schoolteachers. Miss Elizabeth Frere, the first lady superintendent of St John's House, consulted with the Whitelands Training Institute for Schoolmistresses, adopting many of its features such as a modified apprenticeship system with

[31] Williams, 'From Sarah Gamp to Florence Nightingale', p. 69; Summers, 'Pride and Prejudice', p. 35; Dingwall et al., *An Introduction to the Social History of Nursing*, pp. 28–30.

[32] LMA/H01//SJ/A19/1, 7 October 1848.

[33] LMA.H01/ST/SJ/A34/1, 24 May, 2 June 1849.

[34] LMA/H01/ST/SJ/A5/1, 4 June 1849.

[35] CSSJD, Public Meeting 1848, pp. 4–6, 10–13, 16–17.

[36] Ibid., pp. 18–19.

certificates at the end, adequate salaries and living conditions, training in moral and social behaviour, and the goal of improving the social status of the working-class trainees.[37] Finally, from the beginning, St John's House aimed at reforming hospital nursing, and providing a career path for ladies. Fry's organization never planned to reform hospital nursing; its nurses were all working-class women, while the paid superintendents were lower-middle-class women who were not nurses and who were not responsible for the nursing care the nurses gave their patients.

From the time they first started thinking of a training institution, the founders of St John's House planned to have a clergyman, termed the master, as its head. Elizabeth Frere was a charming person of remarkable talent,[38] who gave a great deal of thought to precisely what the master's role should be. She saw three possibilities: making the lady superintendent the supreme authority; placing the lady superintendent under the master, who would be the supreme authority; or the master, lady superintendent and secretary of the council sharing authority equally. It was another indication of Frere's radicalism that she considered placing a clergyman *under* the authority of a lady. In the end, she opted for the master as supreme authority because, after consulting her friends, she found that, as she herself felt, none wished to take the office of lady superintendent without a clergyman with superior authority to support her. The council was a part of the male sphere from which ladies were excluded, therefore ladies could not appear in person at the council. Frere and her friends were not prepared to put themselves in the position of the old matrons, who, like Clementina Cookesley, could face unknown accusations. Ladies, Frere said, would not work under the immediate direction of a group of men because their conduct could be questioned and discussed before a public body at which they could not appear to defend themselves.[39] The authority of the master would become a major issue in only a few years, but in 1849, Frere's decision was pragmatic rather than conservative.

## The Religious Difficulty

The construction of the training school as a religious sisterhood solved the social problem for ladies taking up hospital nursing and conferred respectability on working-class nurses, but it also unfortunately coincided with a climax of religious controversy in mid-nineteenth-century England. The massive immigration of unskilled Catholic Irish labourers who undercut English workers reached its peak during the famine years after 1845, precisely when St John's House was founded. The Irish influx exacerbated long-standing English anti-Catholicism. Many Protestants believed Catholics were superstitious, morally corrupt and a challenge to England's Protestant constitution. The High Church movement's identification

---

[37]    Tropp, *The School Teachers*, pp. 15–22; LMA/H01/ST/SJ/A19/1, 7 October 1848.

[38]    Overton and Wordsworth, *Christopher Wordsworth, Bishop of Lincoln*, pp. 124–5.

[39]    LMA/H01/ST/SJ/A19/1, 1 February 1849.

with the pre-Reformation Church had magnified the fear of Rome, which became worse when a number of high-profile Anglicans converted to Catholicism, most notably John Henry Newman, who took his closest followers with him in 1845, and Henry Edward Manning in 1851. A few of the early Anglican sisterhood superiors converted as well. From the 1840s, the emotional intensity of the debate was heightened by an outpouring of highly salacious 'No Popery' literature. Two favourite themes were sexual relationships between nuns and priests, and young women held prisoners in convents.[40]

Then came the explosive issue popularly known as the Papal Aggression. Since the Reformation, Catholic parishes in Britain were missions governed by vicars apostolic who reported to the Office of Propaganda in Rome. In 1850, to meet the needs of the numerous Irish Catholic immigrants, the Pope created 12 bishops and made the militant Irishman Nicholas Wiseman a cardinal and Archbishop of Westminster. The re-establishment of the Catholic diocesan hierarchy and the presence of an archbishop with a title which was often used as a synonym for Parliament seemed to place the Catholic Church on an equal footing with the Anglican Church and enraged many English people, including Prime Minister Lord John Russell. There was a massive popular outcry and a new wave of virulent anti-Catholicism. The Pope's actions also aroused vicious controversies among Dissenters[41] and within the Anglican Church itself. Because many identified it with Popery, the High Church party now attained the height of its unpopularity; Low Churchmen and Dissenters often formed alliances against the High Church group.[42] Sisterhoods became one of their favourite targets.

**Arrival of Sister Mary Jones**

These violent religious controversies stalled the growth of St John's House, first because many failed to differentiate between Anglican and Catholic sisterhoods, and second because the popular view of hospital nurses as degraded women made both ladies and respectable working-class women reluctant to become probationers. The sisterhood was able to attract experienced hospital nurses, although of those who applied, the Sisters accepted approximately only 1 in 20

---

[40]    Arnstein, *Protestant vs. Catholic in Mid-Victorian England*, pp. 3–4, 6; Chadwick, *The Victorian Church*, vol. 1, pp. 211, 299–300, 271–2, 507.

[41]    Non-Anglican Protestant denominations, such as the Baptists or Congregationalists, were called Dissenters.

[42]    R.J. Schiefen, 'Wiseman, Nicholas Patrick Stephen (1802–1865)', *Oxford Dictionary of National Biography*, <http://www.oxforddnb.com/index/29/101029791> (accessed 10 July 2010); Chadwick, *The Victorian Church*, vol. 1, pp. 275–82, 287–96, 303; D.G. Paz, *Anti-Catholicism in Mid-Victorian England* (Palo Alto, CA, 1992), pp. 6–11; E.R. Norman, *Anti-Catholicism in Victorian England* (New York, 1968), pp. 52–7.

nurses.[43] Like Nightingale at Harley Street, the sisterhood could not recruit enough lady or working-class probationers. Originally, it was hoped working-class probationers would pay a small fee, a kind of apprenticeship payment, but the sisterhood was forced to waive the fee almost immediately because families who could afford to pay preferred to apprentice their daughters to an established trade such as dressmaking or schoolteaching.[44] Mrs Elspeth Morrice, lady superintendent since June 1849, became seriously ill, and the only other resident Sister was Miss Gipps, who acted as lady superintendent during Morrice's frequent periods off sick.[45] The sisterhood was at such a low ebb by 1853 that the council was seriously considering closing it.[46]

On 2 March 1853, a 40-year-old woman named Mary Jones appeared at St John's House asking to become a Sister with a small salary. A week later, Jones returned to make more enquiries about the sisterhood. Two days later, Dr Christopher Wordsworth, later Bishop of Lincoln but then a canon at Westminster Abbey and one of the founders of St John's House, came to the home to speak with Morrice about Jones. The next day, Jones called again, pressing to join the sisterhood. Although Morrice urged the council to accept her as a paid Sister-housekeeper, when the council met on 16 March it refused Jones's request. It was a principle of the sisterhood, the council explained, that the Sisters set an example of Christian humility for the working-class women by working without pay, thus giving dignity to nursing. Two days later, Jones called yet again, accompanied by a Miss Page, possibly the sister of council member Rev. C.W. Page. Then on 28 March 1853, Jones entered the house, not as a Sister, but as the housekeeper with a salary of £20.[47]

Three months later, in June 1853, the council established a committee to decide whether the sisterhood should be disbanded.[48] The committee reported back on 2 July, identifying two principal reasons for the sisterhood's failure to thrive. First, their chaplains had not been effective, resulting in a lack of religious tone and discipline – the two, of course, being synonymous in Victorian thinking. Second, the £50 annual fee which the lady probationers paid to cover the costs of their room and board was a major deterrent for many potential recruits. The committee recommended adjusting the fee to the ability of the individual Sister to pay.[49] Ten days later, on 12 July 1853, Wordsworth called on Morrice and told her that Bishop Blomfield was very anxious to give the sisterhood another year's trial.

43    CSSJD, Annual Reports 1854 and 1855.
44    LMA/H01/ST/SJ/A19/2, 26 May 1849.
45    LMA/H01/ST/SJ/A5/1, 28 July 1851; LMA/H01/ST/SJ/A20/2, 3, and 24 February, 15 March 1853; LMA/H01/ST/SJ/A25.
46    LMA/H01/ST/SJ/A20/2, 17 June 1853.
47    ST/H01/ST/SJ/A2/1, 2, 3 and 16 March 1853; LMA/H01/ST/SJ/A20/2, 3, 9, 11–12, 18 and 28 March 1853; LMA/H01/ST/SJ/A25.
48    LMA/H01/ST/SJ/A20/2, 17 June 1853.
49    CSSJD, Proposed Rules 1848; LMA/H01/ST/SJ/A2/1, 2 July 1853.

As a primary founder of St John's House and president of its council, Blomfield had a real stake in seeing the sisterhood succeed. The council, Wordsworth told Morrice, wished her to resign because her declining health made it impossible for her to fulfil her duties. Morrice resigned on 20 July. Eight days later, Jones gave notice that she was leaving the institution. On 2 August, after a very long meeting suggesting prolonged debate, the council announced that Jones would be received as a Sister with a £20 salary. On 5 August, Wordsworth called again at the home and had a lengthy conversation with Jones.[50] Five days later, the council asked her to be acting lady superintendent, and in November made her permanent superintendent, allowing her to keep her small salary. After another two months, they gave her a £20 gratuity.[51]

Who was Mary Jones? How did she know Miss Page? Did Wordsworth already know her, or was it an intuitive recognition of her extraordinary competence which led him to intervene? Did Jones announce that she was leaving the house on 28 July to force the council to receive her as a Sister and make her acting lady superintendent? What were her family circumstances? We have no answers to these questions. Jones came to St John's House with a recommendation from the Rev. William Armstrong of Brissage. The recommendation has not survived, nor have we been able to track down Armstrong.[52] All that is known about Jones's earlier life[53] is that she was baptized in Tamworth, Staffordshire in December 1812, and her father, Edward Jones, was a cabinet maker,[54] which meant that she was not a lady in the strictest sense of the word, but came from the artisan class. Her father was still alive when she joined St John's House, for she went to spend the day with him in April.[55] She obviously could not rely on him to support her, as she insisted on a salary, the very thing which the council thought made nursing for a lady undignified.

---

[50]   LMA/H01/ST/SJ/A20/2, 12 and 20 July, 2 and 5 August 1853.

[51]   LMA/H01/ST/SJ/A2/1, 10 August, 7 November 1853, 20 February 1854.

[52]   There does not seem to have been a Brissage in England in 1853. There is Brissagio in the Lake District in Italy, where a group of retired Anglican clergy resided. This may explain why Armstrong is not in Crockford's clerical directory, which started a few years later.

[53]   There is a letter from Bishop Blomfield to a Miss Jones, written on 4 February 1848, advising her that there was a sisterhood in London about which he knew very little. He suggested she get in touch with the Rev. W. Dodsworth. (LPA, Blomfield Papers, Microfiches 122–9). This would have been the Park Village Sisterhood. There is no surviving evidence that a Mary Jones ever contacted this sisterhood, and the name Jones, without even a first name, is so common that one cannot assume that this Miss Jones was the Jones of St John's House.

[54]   P. Myers, *Building for the Future: A Nursing History 1896 to 1996* (London, 1996), p. 6.

[55]   LMA/H01/ST/SJ/A20/2, 8 April 1853.

At the same time, Jones was well-educated, spoke good French, and later competently engaged in theological arguments with the Bishop of London.[56] No one, with the sole exception of the master, the Rev. C.P. Shepherd, ever spoke of Jones as being other than a lady. In Shepherd's case, it was not her manners or bearing which he thought disqualified her, but the fact that she accepted a salary.[57] Another indication of her lady-like deportment is that she became one of Nightingale's closest friends, frequently staying at her London home, and also at the Nightingale family homes, Lea Hurst and Embley.[58] Nightingale did not invite any nurse she considered unladylike to her family's homes. The archivist of the sisterhood which Jones later founded never found either a picture of her nor a description of her appearance.[59] One indication that she may not have been physically prepossessing is a comment in 1862 by Henry Bonham Carter, the Secretary of the Nightingale Fund Council. When he first met her, he commented that she did not inspire him with confidence.[60]

From the time she entered St John's House as housekeeper in March 1853, Jones was extremely active. Once appointed lady superintendent, she began advertising for candidates and revising the house rules.[61] Her diary includes medical and nursing details about the nurses and probationers, something Morrice never noted. She appears to have been familiar with medical terminology, so possibly she was already an experienced nurse. Unlike her predecessors Frere and Morrice, she actively nursed at the Westminster and King's College Hospitals. While Morrice seemed oblivious to her nurses' health, Jones showed genuine concern. When Nurse Arnott became too fatigued nursing a private case, Jones brought her home for a night's respite, and only allowed her to return if the family agreed to give her more time for rest. Nurse Rebecca Lawfield returned sick from a case on 6 December 1853. When, a month later, a nurse was requested for an urgent case of bronchitis and pleurisy, Lawfield was the only nurse available. Nevertheless, Jones refused to send her for another two days because she thought she was not yet well enough.[62]

As well, Jones immediately began participating in the larger community. In August and September 1853, she sent night and day nurses to work in the cholera ward at the Westminster Hospital.[63] Then, in 1854 the Crimean War brought

---

[56]   Myers, *Building for the Future*, p. 6; LPA, Tait Papers, vol. 146, fols 3–4; ibid., vol. 148, fols 10–11, 206–7, 214–17.

[57]   LMA/H01/ST/SJ/A25.

[58]   WI/Ms/9001/51 and 76; WI/Ms/9002/101; WI/Ms/9003/64.

[59]   Sister Winifred to Carol Helmstadter, personal communication, St Mary's Convent, London, 1997.

[60]   LMA/H01/ST/A/NFC/73/2.

[61]   LMA/H01/ST/SJ/A20/2, 23 and 24 August, 14 November 1853; LMA/H01/ST/SJ/A2/1, 29 November 1853.

[62]   LMA/H01/ST/SJ/A20/2, 18–19 December 1853, 7 and 9 January 1854.

[63]   LMA/H01/ST/SJ/A20/2, August and September 1853 passim.

nursing to the fore, giving the sisterhood publicity and much improved prospects. Six nurses from St John's House went to Scutari with Florence Nightingale, and St John's House was one of the three organizations which screened and gave brief training to lady volunteers during the war.[64]

## The Struggle for Control of Nursing Practice

At the same time that Jones was training women for the military and naval hospitals serving troops in the Crimean War, the St John's House Council was negotiating with King's College Hospital to provide the larger nursing staff which the hospital would need when it opened a part of its new building.[65] The hospital governors saw four major advantages in turning their nursing over to the sisterhood. First, the moral and religious character of the nurses would be assured; second, the Sisters would establish greater efficiency and improved discipline in the wards; third, the Sisters would stop opportunities for immoral behaviour among the nurses, patients and medical students, and fourth, the governors hoped the Sisters' improvements would attract increased financial contributions from the public.

On the other hand, there were decided disadvantages. First, people might think that because St John's House was a sisterhood it was High Church, and the hospital would suffer from religious prejudice. Second, the governors were concerned by the Sisters' insistence on maintaining control of the nurses rather than placing them, as was standard, under the control of the hospital's committee of management. Finally, there was not yet enough space to accommodate all the nurses within the hospital as St John's House wished. Nevertheless, the committee believed the advantages outweighed these drawbacks.[66]

After long and intricate negotiations, the contract was signed on 1 February, and on 31 March 1856 St John's House began work at King's College Hospital.[67] Jones had won her point of making nursing an autonomous service. The contract specified that members of St John's House must obey all directions from the Hospital Committee, but the nurses no longer reported to that committee, but rather to Lady Superintendent Jones, who in turn reported to the St John's House Council, not the Hospital Committee. St John's House, not the hospital, paid their

---

[64]    The other two training organizations were St Saviour's Home in Osnaburgh Street and an institution established by the Earl of Shaftesbury in Charlotte Street. Taylor, *Eastern Hospitals and English Nurses*, 1st edn, vol. 1, pp. 9–10.

[65]    LMA/H01/ST/SJ/A2/1, 20 October 1854; KH/CM/M4, 9 and 16 February, 9 and 16 March 1855.

[66]    KH/CM/M5, 8 June 1855.

[67]    KH/CM/M5, 3 August 1855, 1 and 8 February, 28 March 1856; LMA/H01/ST/SJ/A2/1, 28 January, 11 February 1856.

nurses, and Jones had complete control of them.[68] This arrangement contrasted sharply with the traditional arrangements for nurses where, as we have seen, hospital committees of management employed, paid and disciplined matrons, assistant nurses and sisters. The autonomy the sisterhood gained also differed markedly from the contract the Nightingale Fund Council signed with St Thomas' Hospital four years later. Under that contract, the Fund paid the hospital for all the probationers' costs, while the hospital's Treasurer and his delegate, Matron Wardroper, who was not a nurse, had complete control of the Nightingale School, including the right to engage and dismiss probationers and nurses and to use probationers as assistant nurses.[69]

Because there was no precedent for the St John's House contract, it was difficult to work out the costs and therefore the amount the hospital should pay the sisterhood. Finally the hospital agreed to provide the nurses' furniture and pay St John's House £800 minus the cost of the nurses' board. When the basement and top stories of the new hospital were finished, they would be assigned to the nurses; until then, the nurses would use the first floor of the old hospital as their residence. The sisterhood would pay for three domestic servants. If St John's House employed more than 20 nurses, they would have to pay for the extra nurses unless the beds in the hospital exceeded 140.[70] The hospital did well to limit its payments to 20 nurses, for Jones soon discovered that she needed more nurses. The contract also specified that, if there was a disagreement between St John's House and the Hospital Committee, it would be submitted to arbitration by the King's College Council.[71] Jones arranged for a sitting room for the nurses, separate bathrooms, and a separate bedroom for each Sister. The nurses slept in dormitories separated by wooden partitions with a curtain at the end, so that each had a small amount of private space. The Sisters and nurses did not have to shop for and cook their own food, but were served their meals in a dining room.[72]

Both Jones and the Master of St John's House, Shepherd, enthusiastically supported the contract with the hospital. Jones thought one of the reasons why the sisterhood had difficulty recruiting Sisters was because it did not offer a well-defined field of labour, such as regular work in a hospital.[73] In addition, she felt it extremely important that St John's House Sisters, rather than the old untrained sisters at the Westminster, St George's or the Middlesex, should train the probationers. The arrangement with King's College Hospital would make this

---

[68]   LMA/H01/ST/SJ/A28/1 (date wrongly given as 1859–64, should be 1855–56); LMA/H01/ST/SJ/A2/1, July 1855–February 1856 passim.

[69]   LMA/H01/ST/A6/13, 10 April 1860.

[70]   LMA/H01/ST/SJ/A2/1. 11 February 1856.

[71]   Ibid.

[72]   Myers, *Building for the Future*, p. 8.

[73]   LMA/H01/ST/SJ/A2/1, 21 April 1855.

possible, and equally important, Jones said, it would fulfil the original overall aim of the sisterhood: to reform hospital nursing.[74]

In February and March 1856 the upcoming contract with the hospital put a great deal of stress on the sisterhood because Jones had to recruit and partially train more probationers within two months. The sisterhood's rule that the lady superintendent defer to the master in all matters of discipline became a major stumbling block. As Jones rapidly tried to build a larger team of probationers, her inability to discharge those whom she found unsuitable – the central problem of the old matrons – brought her into open conflict with Shepherd. His advocacy of the nurses as well as the larger number of probationers led some nurses to become insubordinate. Shepherd attributed their behaviour to what he considered Jones's 'unjust and unmerciful' way of treating them as ordinary servants or overgrown children. He wanted the barrier between the Sisters and the lady superintendent, on the one hand, and the working-class nurses, on the other, gradually withdrawn so that there would be more 'kindly intercourse' between the two classes before the 'great experiment' at King's College Hospital started, and before a 'great, rich, attractive rival institution', presumably the Nightingale Fund Council, formed the previous year, surpassed St John's House.[75]

Jones was indeed a strict disciplinarian. At a meeting with both the lady and the working-class nurses, she reminded them of the importance of obeying the rules. 'And believe me,' she continued:

> I am most fully resolved, for our safety and our credit and our comfort, to have the rules literally obeyed, and that too, willingly and cheerfully. Anything in the shape of disobedience or insubordination shall be instantly repressed. This is only a part of my duty …. Little improprieties, acts of levity and thoughtlessness which, however harmless and perhaps innocent, must be avoided lest the house suffer for the folly of one. I am not reproving any person, I am only seriously exhorting and warning all to be careful, and never to forget that we are by public profession a Christian institution whose character must be maintained by most scrupulous watchfulness.[76]

Significantly, the pages of the lady superintendent's diary from 8 February 1856, shortly after the contract was signed, until March 31, the day the nurses started at King's College Hospital, have been cut out.[77]

Shepherd had been asking for full powers to run the sisterhood since February 1855, when, in what he called the 'interests of efficiency', he asked the council to delegate its authority to one person, namely himself. On this occasion, Jones skilfully blocked Shepherd, telling the council that it must retain its full authority

---

[74]   LMA/H01/ST/SJ/A29.

[75]   LMA/H01/ST/SJ/A24.

[76]   Ibid.

[77]   LMA/H01/ST/SJ/A20/3.

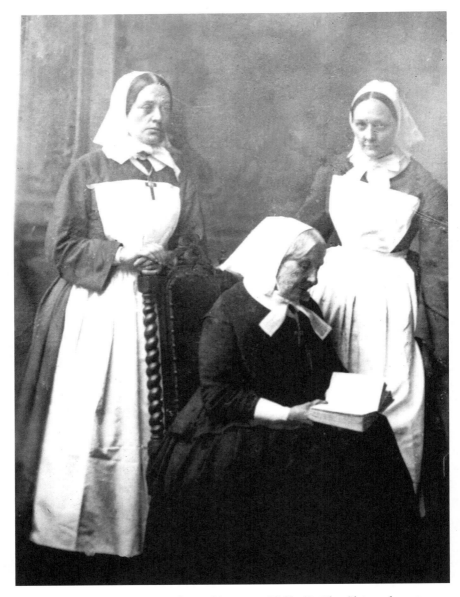

Figure 7.1     Mrs Hodson and two Sisters, *c.* 1868–69. The Sisters do not wear the traditional nuns' habit, but rather the prototype of what was to become the standard nursing uniform: a long-sleeved dress with a bib and apron. The only indication that they are religious Sisters is the cross around their necks.

*Source*: By kind permission of the Trustees of the Guy's and St Thomas' Charity, London.

as a guarantee to the public of the institution's 'soundness of principle and healthiness of action'. She then requested that she be given the power to dismiss nurses. The council refused that request.[78]

When St John's House started work at King's College Hospital, the sisterhood consisted of five resident Sisters and 25 nurses.[79] In addition, there were nineteen Associate Sisters, non-resident ladies who worked part-time helping with recruiting, fundraising and district visiting. After the arrangement with King's College Hospital, these Associate Sisters sometimes worked for months at a time as Sisters in the hospital. Jones took three of the resident Sisters, four of the nurses and four probationers with her to the hospital. Of the two Sisters remaining in the home, Mrs Hodson and Miss Gipps, Jones placed Hodson in charge, although Gipps was her senior. Jones now spent most of her time at the hospital, where Hodson also frequently helped.[80]

On 9 May 1856, following a disagreement between Jones and Shepherd, the details of which are not recorded, the council finally gave Jones sole control of the nurses with power to dismiss them; nurses could no longer appeal to the master to reverse her decisions.[81] The consolidation of authority in the lady superintendent led to the Sisters' system of nursing becoming known as the 'central system', as opposed to the decentralized ward system.

Jones had won her point, but Shepherd did not give up easily. A month later, Jones and Gipps were at odds, with Shepherd strongly supporting Gipps. He was infuriated by the way Jones called him in as a support for her authority, giving him no opportunity to investigate whether the nurse was in the right or the wrong. She had, he said, absolutely no intention of accepting instructions from him. In fact, she was often heard to say that the very title 'master' was a mistake. Shepherd thought Jones caused the disciplinary problems herself by setting an example of disobedience to him.[82] He believed the nurses loved and respected Gipps and disliked Jones. He, Morrice and Gipps had supported the appointment of Jones as the paid housekeeper in 1853, but when the council made Jones lady superintendent, raising her from Gipps's servant to Gipps's mistress, 'the evils which might have been anticipated' began. Shepherd believed Jones's parvenu social position made her insecure, jealous and hostile towards her former mistress. Gipps had been on sick leave since February, and Shepherd thought that as more Sisters joined the sisterhood, Jones was recruiting them to her faction and they planned to push Gipps out when she returned.[83]

Shepherd correctly identified the central issue in the dispute, the issue over which Frere had cogitated. As he succinctly put it: was the lady superintendent under the direction of the master, 'where the law of nature places him, *over* and not *under* any

---

[78] LMA/H01/ST/SJ/A26/1; LMA/H01/ST/SJ/A2/1, 26 February, 21 April 1855.
[79] LMA/H01/ST/SJ/A29.
[80] LMA/H01/ST/SJ/A20/3, April–June 1856 passim; KH/CM/M5, 25 July 1856.
[81] LMA/H01/ST/SJ/A2/1, 9 May 1856.
[82] LMA/H01/ST/SJ/A26/3.
[83] LMA/H01/ST/SJ/A25; LMA/H01/ST/SJ/A26/2.

female officer', or was the master under the direction of the lady superintendent?[84] For Shepherd, St John's House 'was an artificial family with the master as its head or father'. The alteration in the rules giving Jones complete control of the nurses in effect abolished the position of master. 'It is also the first step', Shepherd wrote, 'in a course of policy which must terminate in substituting a woman for a man in the government of the house: a result which the master believes, would speedily leave no house to be governed'.[85]

Shepherd had been an active and energetic chaplain, but his wish to supplant the council as the executive authority had not made him popular with them. The council unanimously supported Jones, finding insufficient grounds for Shepherd's allegations. In June the Council asked him to resign, but he refused. Jones had apparently threatened to resign if Shepherd were allowed to continue as master, for Shepherd complained he was being victimized because some council members were frightened by her threat to resign. In July 1856 Shepherd finally resigned, and in October Gipps followed suit.[86]

Besides breaking what Shepherd and most men of his time considered a law of nature, Jones was now appearing in person at the council meetings – a major breakthrough into the male sphere.[87] Even Jane Nelson, the much-respected matron of the London Hospital, could only report to her committee of management in writing. Did Jones seize the master's executive authority because she was searching for a position of power for herself, as many would later accuse the Anglican Sisters of doing? Or was it primarily that, without a centralized system and the necessary authority to establish good discipline among her nurses, she, like the old matrons, simply could not run an effective nursing system? Shepherd believed the former interpretation. Jones's own writings, although not mentioning this particular incident, support the latter – she could not run an efficient nursing service without the requisite authority. Radical action, including breaking commonly accepted gender barriers, was needed to achieve efficiency in hospital nursing.

**Conclusion**

Jones had succeeded in centralizing responsibility for nursing in the lady superintendent, and could now start work developing the new nursing service at King's College Hospital. It would be the beginning of a major reform in nursing: the establishment of a system which in 1874 the *British Medical Journal* would describe as 'the best system of nursing yet introduced'.[88] In the next chapter, we

[84]  LMA/H01/ST/ SJ/A26/4 (original emphases).
[85]  LMA/H01/ST/SJ/A26/2.
[86]  LMA/H01/ST/SJ/A2/1, 9 and 23 June, 21 October 1856; LMA/H01/ST/ SJ/A35/1, 18 June 1856.
[87]  LMA/H01/ST/SJ/A2/1, 7 July 1856.
[88]  *BMJ*, 4 April 1874, p. 461.

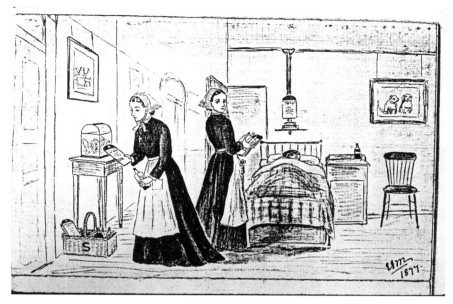

Figure 7.2    Lady probationers in Sambrooke Ward, King's College Hospital,
              1877. The lady probationers wear crosses but are secular nurses, not
              necessarily in training to be religious Sisters. Note the efforts to give
              the ward a home-like feeling: the goldfish and pictures on the wall.
              In the wealthier hospitals there were often Oriental rugs on the floor,
              and always plants.

*Source*: By kind permission of the Community of St John the Divine, Birmingham.

look at the way the St John's House Sisters and the All Saints Sisters' reforms
played out in the three London hospitals where they held the contracts, and the
work of the British Nursing Association, an evangelical group which introduced
the Sisters' central system at the Royal Free Hospital. What explains the dramatic
success of the central nursing system?

# Chapter 8
# The St John's House
# Central Nursing System

### The Contract at King's College Hospital

Sister Mary Jones had gained control of the nursing service at King's College Hospital and was now able to develop a training system which she and her Sisters directed. At mid-century, ladies, with their superior education and 'command', as Nightingale put it, were essential for organizing and directing the barely literate working-class nurses. When St John's House was founded, the expectation had been that the head nurses would be exclusively the religious Sisters, because they were ladies. Nevertheless, it was not a mistress–servant relationship, as has sometimes been suggested.[1] As we have noted, the upper-middle-class Sisters had the same clinical training as the paid working-class nurses. Even before the training institution opened, the council and Elizabeth Frere were not prepared to make ladies head nurses unless they had specific training in nursing. Frere told the council in 1848 that it was essential to offer the working-class nurses a good salary 'to attract the best sort', because St John's House needed to have the best instructors for the probationers.[2] Until 1856, lady as well as working-class probationers took direction from working-class hospital sisters under whom they were placed for their clinical experience. Furthermore, the training the working-class probationers received was aimed at improving their social status, not establishing a mistress–servant relationship.[3] By 1861, Jones was planning to make able working-class nurses, after a five-year probation, sisters in the sense of head nurses.[4]

Jones was a strict disciplinarian, as we have seen, but despite Shepherd's attestations to the contrary, she and her Sisters were very supportive of their nurses. Jones appreciated that it was the system rather than the nurses themselves which caused so many of the nurses' failings. 'We have left the poor Hospital nurse as the victim of a vicious system,' Jones wrote to Nightingale, '& then condemn and shrink from her as degraded.'[5] She thought a lady superintendent

---

[1]   Summers, *Angels and Citizens*, pp. 21–2; Dingwall et al., *An Introduction to the Social History of Nursing*, pp. 41–2, 47.

[2]   LMA/H01/ST/SJ/A19/1, 7 October 1848.

[3]   LMA/H01/ST/SJ/A17/1; cf. Summers, 'Ministering Angels', pp. 142, 144–5.

[4]   BL 47743, fol. 86.

[5]   BL 47743, fol. 202.

should have a 'mother's feeling for, and sympathy with her nurses'.[6] She should be 'a large hearted, loving Christian woman, clear-sighted & firm – but forbearing & patient'.[7] When Jones and her Sisters left St John's House in 1868, the Sister who replaced her at King's said that if Jones were to accept a position in another hospital, which in fact she did not, all the nurses would immediately leave and follow her there.[8]

The Sisters' supportive approach is well illustrated by an event during the Crimean War. At Scutari, the six working-class St John's House nurses were appalled when Nightingale, her matron Mary Clarke, and her friend and chaperone Selina Bracebridge, treated them in the conventional manner, revealing their sense of social superiority and deep-seated distrust of working-class women. One nurse wrote to Jones: 'Miss Nightingale treats us with disrespect and unkindness.' Another reported they had been treated with contempt ever since Shepherd, who had accompanied them to Paris, had left them. She regretted they had come out 'without someone to care for us'. A third, Elizabeth Drake, also wished 'most earnestly' that someone from home were there to care for them. The St John's House nurses never got a kind word, she told Jones, but Drake was more distressed by the way they were distrusted. 'We do not look for many comforts,' she wrote, 'but we do feel we ought to be trusted.'[9]

Of the six St John's House nurses, Nightingale considered Drake invaluable, and Rebecca Lawfield an unskilful nurse who did not know a fractured limb when she saw one, but nevertheless valuable because of her propriety and kindness. Nightingale asked Jones to recall the other four because their manners were so 'flibberty-gibbet' and they did not observe the rules she had made to preserve female decorum. They fed the men without medical orders, their dressings were careless and slovenly, and they would not take orders from anyone except Nightingale herself.[10]

Jones sent Nightingale a letter of recall for the four nurses, which she told Nightingale she could either use or withhold as she saw fit. Nightingale's superior social position did not intimidate Jones, for she then went on to tell Nightingale that she had received letters from three of the nurses complaining that they were being treated with disrespect and were not being used to good effect. She had laid the letters before the St John's House council and its president, Bishop Blomfield. All shared Jones's regret that the nurses had gone to Scutari 'unaccompanied by someone from home to whom they could have looked for kind counsel in obeying your rules and carrying out your orders'. She regretted that Nightingale had used:

---

6   BL 47744, fols 134–5.
7   BL 47743, fol. 80.
8   WI/Ms/9003/19.
9   LMA/H01/ST/NC3/SU12–13, 15–16.
10   LMA/H01/ST/NC3/SU14.

expressions which would seem to betoken a want of consideration towards women who volunteered to aid in carrying out, under your control and guidance, a good though difficult and arduous work on an hitherto untried field of labour. Mrs Drake, for whom I share your high regard, is very unhappy and feels much hurt that she is not allowed to be so useful as she might be expected to be and that her anxiety and that of her sister nurses should be turned to a wrong account.

Jones did not know what to make of the accusation of 'flibberty-gibbet' behaviour; she did not think flighty and frivolous behaviour was characteristic of her four nurses. She had impressed on them before they left London that they were to obey no one except Nightingale, and suggested that perhaps they had taken this instruction too literally. Regarding the want of skill to diagnose a fracture, Jones could only say that St John's House trained women to be nurses, not surgeons.[11]

As well as the need to treat nurses with respect, Jones insisted on the need for nursing knowledge. She deplored the idea that two or three months' training was adequate. When she came to St John's House, three months' training was the general rule; she extended it to a whole year.[12] As well as clinical experience in the hospitals during the day, the training included religious instruction from Jones and the chaplain every evening. As well, Jones gave simple lessons on the structure and functions of the body, designed to increase the nurses' interest in their work and strengthen their clinical efficiency.[13] By 1863, a two-year probation was necessary for those who were going to teach nursing.[14] 'Why will not people think it necessary to be well and fully prepared for what they undertake,' Jones complained in 1867, 'instead of only hurriedly skimming the surface of that knowledge which they need for the undertaking?'[15] She refused to take ladies for a month or two of training; she had a horror 'of turning an army of half taught nurses loose among the sick poor'.[16] Unlike the Nightingale School, which into the 1890s continued to accept probationers throughout the year when assistant nurse positions became vacant, Jones organized the classes and lectures on a term system, and accepted probationers only at the beginning of the term.[17] The Sisters gave classes and instruction in the manual work of a nurse, and doctors gave lectures on medical subjects.[18] Like Nightingale, Jones was convinced that a

[11]  LMA/H01/ST/NC3/SU17.

[12]  BL 47743, fols 88–91, 131–4, 141–6.

[13]  LMA/H01/NC/16/5, p. 20.

[14]  BL 47743, fols 197–9.

[15]  BL 47744, fols 101–2.

[16]  BL 47743, fols 88–91. Jones agreed, for Nightingale's sake, to make an exception for Agnes Jones, but she had spent seven months at Kaiserswerth and also trained at St Thomas'.

[17]  For St Thomas', see, BL 47739, fols 101, 246; BL 47740, fols 85–6, 106–7. For Jones, see, BL 47743, fol. 200; BL 47744, fols 24–8.

[18]  Ibid., fols 59–61.

public hospital with a medical school, despite 'all its difficulties & disagreements, is the only school for a sound & healthy training of nurses – whether gentlewomen or others'.[19]

Jones herself made a point of keeping up with current practice and professional issues. Her diary and correspondence reveal regular and varied activities. When the negotiations for the contract with King's College Hospital were in process, she and two Sisters visited St Bartholomew's, and Mrs Hodson and another Sister went to Guy's. When the Nightingale Fund was launched in November 1855, Jones and two Sisters attended the meeting.[20] In November 1860, Jones and three Sisters went to the opening of the Statistical Congress at King's College, and two days later Jones and Mrs Hodson went to a lecture on sanitary architecture at the South Kensington Museum.[21] In 1865, Jones visited Paris and inspected hospitals there, using an introduction from Nightingale to the director general of all the Paris hospitals.[22]

Jones was not an enthusiast for ladies' nursing. She told Nightingale that she was sick of 'the babble about ladies' work'. Talk about nursing was so sentimental, she grumbled, 'The nonsense one hears daily is hard to bear.'[23] She thought Miss Soden, the lady superintendent at the Bath United Hospital, made the common mistake of trying to find 'lady's work' in hospitals, rather than having ladies accept the hospitals as they were and improving them. Jones designed the sisterhood for the work, rather than finding suitable work for ladies. Work, such as scrubbing and drudgery that was unsuitable for ladies, she asserted, was unsuitable for any nurse. If the hospital was not fit for lady nurses, it was not fit for any women. In classic Victorian terms, Jones explained, 'True refinement and purity' would only make a woman more fit to take such a work in hand and make hospital nursing what it ought to be.[24]

While Jones exhibited Victorian pieties with her sense of true refinement and purity, she was extremely practical in her approach to nursing reform. To have a nursing system that worked smoothly, she argued, it was always better to send a team of nurses who had been trained in the same method, rather than sending one nurse here and another there. Instead of building a new hospital, it made more sense to take over an existing general hospital, work it well, and train nurses there for teaching in other institutions. She emphasized the importance of working with management and making changes gradually. She advocated being patient but firm: it took time for things to dovetail and work smoothly. She thought it pointless to ask a governor to surrender his authority to someone else, and when a new nursing

[19]   BL 47743, fol. 179.
[20]   LMA/H01/ST/SJ/A20/3, 27 and 29 November, 4 December 1855.
[21]   LMA/H01/ST/SJ/A20/5, 16 and 18 July 1860.
[22]   LMA/H01/ST/ST/NC1/65/11 and 12.
[23]   BL 47743, fols 178–80, 202; BL 47744, fols 138–9.
[24]   BL 47743, fols 178–80, 202.

system started, it was to be expected that initially, governors would be jealous and fearful for their authority. But, she said, 'that will wear off'.[25]

In order to make hospitals run more efficiently, it was first necessary to determine the causes of the difficulties. Jones did not believe that busy doctors were in a position to do that; in fact, she sometimes thought they were indifferent to it.[26] Here, she put her finger on one of the central problems of the ward system. Some doctors were genuinely interested in improving the nursing, but most senior men only visited their wards two or three times a week, and were not prepared to devote the amount of time which John Flint South, for example, gave to educating his sisters.

Jones told Nightingale that sisterhoods were the only reliable agencies for nursing hospitals and workhouse infirmaries. The Sisters had:

> all the manual skill – knowledge & common sense of the best secular nurses – and a great deal more besides. I know well you do not quite agree . but I feel quite sure dearest friend, that, were you now actively employed ... personally engaged in the actual nursing of Hospitals etc – you would, you must – come to the same conclusion.[27]

Finally, Jones wished to advance the cause of women. She wanted to help 'any willing & capable women to have, & to fulfil, some useful object in life'. No trouble should be spared to achieve this end. She admired the example Nightingale was setting for her fellow women — and also men. 'May it [Nightingale's example] arouse & strengthen many,' she concluded.[28]

The sisterhood flourished under Jones's guidance. In 1855–56, 25 private nurses earned £590; in 1863–64, 40 private nurses earned £1,877. In 1855–56, usually 5 out of the 25 nurses were unemployed; in 1863–64, all the nurses were employed as far as their health and strength permitted, and demand exceeded the supply. The sisterhood was doing more work with the sick poor than ever before, and together with the Nightingale Fund, had established a midwifery school at King's College Hospital. The Sisters were also training women for district nursing.[29]

At the end of the Sisters' first year at King's College Hospital, its governors expressed their appreciation of 'the gentleness, intelligence, affection, untiring zeal and self-denial' of the lady superintendent, lady sisters and nurses.[30] Jones's improvements, however, were expensive. The hospital's female staff before she took over consisted of 28 women: 15 nurses, ten part-time scrubbers, a cook,

[25]   BL 47744, fols 11–12, 37–8.
[26]   BL 47743, fols 81–2.
[27]   BL 47744, fol. 91.
[28]   BL 47743, fols 96, 148.
[29]   LMA/H01/ST/SJ/A29.
[30]   LMA/H01/ST/SJ/A8/1.

a kitchen maid and a housemaid.[31] Jones brought seven nurses and four probationers with her on 31 March, and five of the old nurses chose to stay on, making a total of 17 nurses, counting Jones herself. By July 1856 there were four Sisters plus a probationary Sister, 15 nurses and ten probationers, plus two more training for district nursing, and Jones – 33 nurses all living in the hospital. Jones laid off the part-time scrubbers and hired five domestic servants, three for the hospital and two to look after the St John's House nurses,[32] making a total female staff of 38. Jones had more than doubled the number of nurses – from 15 to 33. No other hospital in England in 1856 offered such good living and staffing conditions. However, there was a serious drawback to Jones's enhanced nursing service: it cost far more than either the hospital or St John's House had anticipated.

King's College Hospital was no longer understaffed, but from a financial point of view, the larger, better-trained staff boomeranged because the better the nursing, the more sophisticated medicine and surgery the doctors could practice, and hence the more nurses they needed. The contract had posited nurses for 120 beds, but three months after the Sisters took over, 134 beds were in use and the hospital planned to open six more.[33] At the end of the first year, St John's House had spent £1,635 6s. 5d. – that is, £835 more than the hospital was paying.[34] The council renegotiated the contract, but King's was one of the least well endowed hospitals, and while the governors fully recognized the superiority of the Sisters' nursing, they could afford only £300 more for the next year. St John's House could not afford to continue subsidizing the hospital at that rate. Yet the Sisters felt they could not decrease their expenditure without decreasing the quality of nursing care. Their council therefore launched a fundraising drive.[35] By 1883, King's was paying £3,579 for a staff of 69 nurses nursing 205 beds – an amount which meant the sisterhood was still subsidizing the hospital.[36]

### The Contract with Charing Cross

In 1866, Jones negotiated a similar contract with Charing Cross Hospital. She obtained improved sleeping accommodation for the nurses by moving the resident medical officer and the chaplain out of their rooms and giving them to the nurses.[37] Three months after St John's House began work at Charing Cross, the governors expressed their appreciation of the improvement in the nursing. The much-changed and improved appearance of the wards spoke for itself, they said. The Sisters were:

[31]  KH/CM/M4, 27 January 1854.
[32]  KH/CM/M5, 25 July 1856.
[33]  Ibid.
[34]  LMA/H01/ST/SJ/A2/1, 24 November 1857.
[35]  LMA/H01/ST/SJ/A2/1, 15 April, 4 May 1858.
[36]  LMA/H01/ST/SJ/A39.
[37]  CCH/WB, 13 November 1866; CCH/MBG, 3 July 1865.

very experienced, and being educated ladies, are competent and properly prepared to carry out with exactness and judgment the instructions they receive from the medical men. They are by habit fully qualified to govern others and to see that the nurses – all of whom are carefully selected – do their duty faithfully and kindly.[38]

The governors' attribution of the Sisters' success to their social status and experience as household managers rather than to their skilled nursing practice, their improved working conditions or their nurses' training would become the generally held view both then and now.[39] This perception supported the mystique which earlier historians conferred on lady nurses, whom they saw as the chief agents of nineteenth-century nursing reform.[40] While the Sisters' experience working with domestic staffs, their superior education and their social position in a deferential society contributed to their success, these factors were less important than their nursing expertise and their approach to their nurses and patients. Their *esprit de corps*, which the doctors so admired, and their efforts to make hospital nursing 'a respectable, desirable employment',[41] as Jones described it, were two other keys to their success.

## The Central System at University College Hospital

St John's House was the primary inspiration for the nursing services at two other London teaching hospitals: University College Hospital and the Royal Free Hospital. The long association of the All Saints Sisters of the Poor with University College Hospital began in December 1859, when Harriet Brownlow Byron, the Mother Foundress, asked the hospital's committee of management to allow two Sisters to come to the hospital to learn how to nurse and dress wounds.[42] This Anglican community was a very High Church sisterhood founded in 1851. The Sisters cared for aged women, incurables and orphans, ran a crèche for working mothers in their home on Margaret Street, and also did school and district work.[43]

Byron, together with another Sister, had had what was then considered training as a nurse at King's College Hospital in 1855.[44] In 1859, Byron taught

---

[38]    CCH/MBG, 28 February 1867.

[39]    See, for example, Dingwall et al., *An Introduction to the Social History of Nursing*, p. 29.

[40]    Dock and Stewart, *A Short History of Nursing*, pp. 113–14, 126; Tooley, *The History of Nursing in the British Empire*, pp. 83–4.

[41]    BL 47743, fols 11–12.

[42]    UCH/A1/2/2, 21 December 1859.

[43]    Mayhew, *All Saints*, pp. 32–3.

[44]    KH/CM/M4, 2 February 1855.

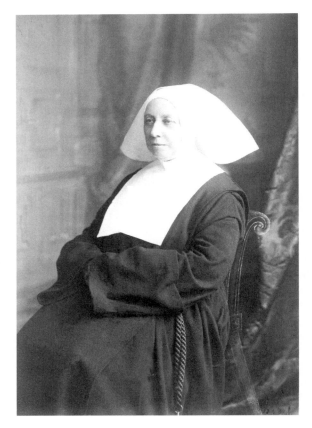

Figure 8.1     Mother Foundress Harriet Brownlow Byron. The traditional nun's
               habit which Byron wears illustrates how it was impossible, from
               simply looking at them, to tell the difference between the Anglican
               and Roman Catholic Sisters.

*Source*: By kind permission of the Society of the All Saints Sisters of the Poor, Oxford.


Outside Sister[45] (later Mother) Caroline Mary how to do dressings in the All Saints
Home. Sister Caroline Mary handed Byron the lint and ointment for the dressings,
which Byron applied skilfully and gently, using forceps, not her fingers. Byron
also taught her how to bandage with hot, wrung-out flannels and how to cut a large
blister. Sister Caroline Mary and another Sister then went to University College
Hospital as observers, following the dressers and nurse from bed to bed as they

---

[45]   Outside Sisters were the equivalent of the St John's House Associate Sisters,
women who lived at home and worked part-time with the community.

dressed wounds.[46] The two Sisters' training by observing the dressers and nurses, probably only for a few weeks, is typical of what was considered an appropriate training for ladies at most hospitals well into the 1870s.[47]

In 1860, when a head nurse in charge of two wards at University College Hospital resigned after being reprimanded for misconduct, Byron suggested that an All Saints Sister replace her.[48] The hospital agreed, and appropriately on All Saints Day, St John's House-trained Sister Elizabeth and three women from the All Saints Home whom she planned to train as nurses took over the two wards. Sister Elizabeth soon had the wards in what Sister Caroline Mary remembered as good 'order, comfort and refinement'.

In September 1861, following a serious railroad accident at Camden Town, 30–40 injured passengers were brought to University College Hospital. Fifteen were put in Sister Elizabeth's wards, where, because she could get extra help from other Sisters at the All Saints Home, she was able to give them excellent care. The doctors were very impressed, and urged the governors to extend the Sisters' contract to the whole hospital.[49] Although some governors had serious reservations about delegating so much authority to a High Church organization, the hospital decided to give the Sisters the contract. As at St John's House, the Sisters worked gratis and Sisters and nurses were directly responsible to the mother superior, not the hospital committee. The hospital originally paid the sisterhood £1,000 a year for their services but, as did St John's House, the Sisters had to refund the cost of the food for their staff.[50] Also as at St John's House, the Sisters soon found they needed more nurses, and by 1863 the nursing was costing them more than the hospital paid.[51]

On 2 June 1862 the Sisters moved into the remaining hospital wards. There was 'mess and confusion' everywhere, and 'the patients utterly neglected and everything most dirty and untidy', Sister Caroline Mary recalled. Sir William Jenner, physician-extraordinary to Queen Victoria and considered the leading consultant of his day,[52] told her the 'gamps, bad nurses' drank the patients'

---

[46]   ASA, Mother Caroline Mary Box, 'Memories of Sister Caroline Mary', pp. 2–3, 7–8; ASA, 'U.C.H.', UCH Box.

[47]   See, for example, LMA/H02/WH/A1/42, 4 February 1868; LMA/H02/WH/A1/44, 13 February, 23 April 1872; SM/AD1/11, 25 February, 22 July 1870, 13 January, 16 June 1871; SM/AD1/13, 19 March, 15 October 1875, 11 February 1876; see also E.A. Beaufort, Viscountess Strangford, *Hospital Training for Ladies* (London, 1874), pp. 10–14.

[48]   W.R. Merrington, *University College Hospital and its Medical School: A History* (London, 1976), p. 251; UCH/A1/2/2, 1 August 1860.

[49]   ASA, Mother Caroline Mary Box, 'Memories', pp. 2–3, 7–8; ASA, UCH Box 'U.C.H.'; UCH/A1/2/2, 1 August, 10 and 24 October 1860.

[50]   UCH/A1/2/2, 29 January, 12 and 26 March, 9 and 23 April, 1862.

[51]   UCH/A1/2/2, 4 November 1863.

[52]   W.I. McDonald, 'Jenner, Sir William, first baronet (1815–1898)', *Oxford Dictionary of National Biography*, <www.oxforddnb.com/view/article/14754> (accessed 10 July 2011).

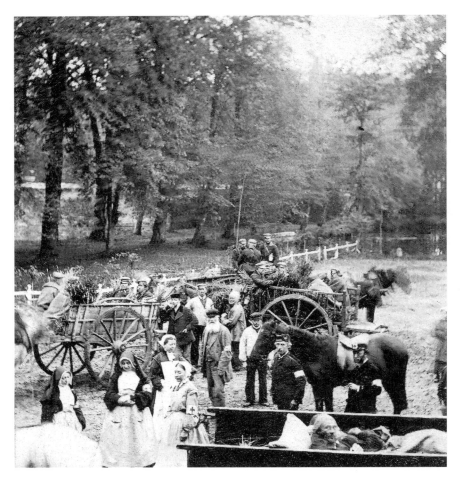

Figure 8.2     All Saints Sisters and an Anglo-American ambulance in the Franco–
Prussian War, 1870–71. 'Ambulance' in the nineteenth century
meant a mobile hospital as well as the wooden wagon in which the
wounded are being conveyed here.

*Source*: By kind permission of the Society of the All Saints Sisters of the Poor, Oxford.

stimulants and caroused with the men patients and porters at night. The Sisters
dismissed all the old nurses and started afresh with their own staff. The hospital
assigned its top floor to the Sisters for their cells, community room, refectory and
oratory. The probationers lived in the All Saints Home, going to the hospital every
day at 9 a.m. and returning to the Home after supper in time for Compline. As at
St John's House, the Sisters rotated probationers through the wards, but they did
make some significant modifications to the central system. Their assistant nurses

did a good deal of the cleaning,[53] and there are not the frequent discussions of training issues found in the St John's House records. Nevertheless, the Sisters gave classes, and by at least the 1880s doctors were giving the nurses lectures. In 1862 the training was only for one year, but by the 1870s it was two, and by the 1890s three years.[54]

Despite some complaints from the doctors about rotating nurses through the hospital, the Sisters' apprenticeship system was overall very successful. At the University College Hospital Annual Dinner in 1869, Sir William Jenner and Mr Enfield, the Treasurer, spoke of the immense improvement in the nursing. Despite the prejudice against High Church sisterhoods, they said, the Sisters' nursing system had gained the highest praise from people of all creeds; that praise was the best argument against theoretical objections made by those who preferred the old ways.[55] In 1870–71, seven Sisters under the direction of Byron nursed in the Franco–Prussian War, where the doctors considered them a top-class team.[56]

Although their contracts were less progressive than those of St John's House, the All Saints Sisters brought the same kind of religious discipline and service to the sick poor, and the same sense of Christian nurture which enabled them to recruit and retain nurses and to provide first-class nursing care.

Speaking primarily of Catholic Sisters, Sioban Nelson concluded that nursing emerged as 'a hybrid religious and professional practice'.[57] This was indeed true of the Catholic nursing Sisters, who made it a part of their nursing duties to care for their patients' spiritual welfare.[58] Some modern nursing historians have assumed that the Anglican Sisters likewise tried to save their patients' souls.[59] Many of the Sisters' contemporaries thought the same thing, but this perception was entirely wrong. The contracts with King's College and Charing Cross Hospitals placed the chaplains in sole charge of spiritual ministrations; St John's House agreed not to interfere in any religious matter.[60] Similarly, before the All Saints Sisters entered University College Hospital, their mother superior assured the hospital governors that her Sisters would not interfere with the religious opinions of the hospital's

[53]   UCH/A1/2/2, 23 April 1862; ASA, Mother Caroline Mary Box, 'Memories of Sister Caroline Mary', pp. 8–9, 19.

[54]   UCH/A1/2/2, 22 October 1862; UCH/A1/2/6, 28 October 1885; J. Likeman, *Nursing at University College Hospital, London 1862–1948* (London, 2002), p. 154.

[55]   *Lancet*, 26 June 1869, p. 885. See also *Lancet*, 16 July 1870, p. 100.

[56]   ASA, Mother Foundress Box, 'Diary of Franco-Prussian War', pp. 1, 97–8.

[57]   Nelson, *Say Little, Do Much*, pp. 5–6.

[58]   See, for example, Bridgeman, 'An Account', pp. 177–8.

[59]   Dingwall et al., *An Introduction to the Social History of Nursing*, pp. 28–30; A. Summers, 'The Costs and Benefits of Caring: Nursing Charities c. 1830–c.1860', in J. Barry and C. Jones (eds), *Medicine and Charity Before the Welfare State* (London, 1991), pp. 138–9.

[60]   CCH/MBG, 28 February 1867.

officers, servants or patients.[61] In the older teaching hospitals such as Guy's, the ward sister was supposed to read prayers daily and the assistant nurses were ordered to 'endeavour by their example to enforce on the Patients the necessity of attention to the duties of Religion'. All patients who were well enough were required to attend morning prayers in the chapel. By contrast, the All Saints Sisters said no prayers in the wards[62] and did no religious counselling. Although both the All Saints and the St John's House Sisters personally believed they were serving Christ when they nursed the sick poor, and while their Christian commitment and values were obvious to their patients and colleagues, their nursing practice was entirely secular.

## The Central System at the Royal Free Hospital

If the All Saints' Sisters' nursing service was a High Church version of the Broad Church St John's House system, the British Nursing Association (BNA)[63] was an evangelical form of it. In 1867 a group of devout army officers, led by Major General Sir Arthur Lawrence and his wife, established this association, originally known as the London Training School and Home for Nurses. It began very much as had St John's House, working in private homes, hospitals and among the sick poor, and sending probationers as day pupils to different hospitals for training.[64]

In September 1867 the BNA concluded an agreement with St Mary's Hospital to train six women who would reside in the hospital as probationers. In January 1868 the BNA increased the number to eight, and in April 1869 added four non-resident probationers.[65] By December 1869 the BNA had acquired a lady superintendent, Miss Louisa E.C. Coles, and a nurses' home in Paddington near the hospital. Coles wanted all the probationers to live in the home, where she could provide moral tutelage and give theoretical instruction which, she said, made nurses more interested in their work. The hospital asked that all probationers be resident, and was unhappy with Coles's visits to her probationers on the wards. The governors thought she interfered with the working of the hospital, while Coles was dissatisfied with her limited ability to clinically supervise her

[61]   UCH A1/2/2, 3 August, 21 December 1859.

[62]   LMA/H09/GY/ A53/1, pp. 95, 101; LMA/H09/GY/A71/1, p. 677; LMA/A/ NFC/22/4, p. 31; Likeman, *Nursing at University College Hospital, London*, pp. 44–5.

[63]   Despite the similarity in names, the British *Nursing* Association had nothing to do with the British *Nurses* Association which Ethel Bedford Fenwick founded in 1887.

[64]   BL 45759, fols 110–12, 116–17, 120, 127–8, 152, 175.

[65]   F.A. Eardley-Wilmot, *Memorials of Frederick M. Eardley-Wilmot: Major-General Royal Artillery and Fellow of the Royal Society* (London, 1879), p. 179; SM/AD/7/4, 7 August, 22 December 1869; LMA/H09/GY/A67/4/1, 17 March 1869, 16 February 1870.

probationers. However, the hospital gave in when General Lawrence insisted that the probationers live in the BNA's home.[66]

At this time the Royal Free Hospital was becoming increasingly dissatisfied with its nursing. In July 1868 the governors transferred official responsibility for the nurses from the matron to the house surgeon, and in November the doctors established a medical committee which began mooting the question of training nurses in the hospital.[67] When at the end of January 1870 Colonel Pitcairn, the BNA's Honorary Secretary, sent the governors information about the BNA, they leapt at the opportunity to secure its nursing. They met with Pitcairn and Coles in February, and signed a contract in early March.[68] The BNA withdrew its nurses from St Mary's in May 1870, and began work at the Royal Free in June.[69] General Eardley Wilmot, a life-long friend of Lawrence and a BNA board member, then joined the hospital board.[70]

The Royal Free contract was modelled on the sisterhoods' contracts. It allowed the BNA to train probationers in the hospital as long as they did not increase hospital costs. The BNA provided 18 nurses for the six wards in the hospital; each ward had one efficient nurse, defined as having six months or more instruction, one certified (that is fully trained) nurse and one night nurse. Nurses and probationers were not to scrub floors or clean grates. The hospital paid £276 a year, and provided board, accommodation and washing for the lady superintendent and 15 of the 18 nurses. The BNA paid for the laundry and board of the remaining three. A year later, the BNA had added two more nurses to the hospital staff.[71] As did the sisterhoods, the BNA was subsidizing the hospital, and would continue to do so for its 14-year stay there. Similarly, as the better nursing enabled medical activity to increase and as the hospital expanded its space, the number of nurses and their costs kept increasing. By 1878 there were 29 nurses plus the lady superintendent, at an annual cost of £625.[72]

Using the Nightingale School curriculum, the BNA gave its probationers formal instruction; both the house surgeon and the lady superintendent held classes. Lady probationers could attend for as little as three months at a guinea a week, but unless they had previous training, most opted for the full year term which was required of ordinary probationers. Coles gave certificates only after one year of service.[73]

Coles was generally a success, although, as at University College Hospital, there were occasional complaints that the nurses were changed too often and that

[66]  SM/AD1/11, 16 December 1869; LMA/A/NFC/22/4, pp. 56–7.
[67]  RFH/WB, 16 July, 5 November 1868, 8 and 15 July 1869.
[68]  RFH/WB, 27 January, 3 and 24 February, 10 March 1870.
[69]  SM/AD1/11, 20 May 1870; RFH/A6, p. 11.
[70]  Eardley-Wilmot, *Memorials of Frederick M. Eardley-Wilmot*, pp. 192–3.
[71]  RFH/WB, 24 February, 10 March 1870; 12 October 1871.
[72]  RFH/WB, 7 March 1878.
[73]  LMA/A/NFC/22/4, pp. 32–5.

inadequately trained probationers were sometimes used as efficient nurses.[74] On arrival, Coles arranged for a short service on Sunday mornings for the probationers and patients. Like Jones, she insisted on a housemaid to clean the nurses' quarters, wait at table, wash up after meals, and clean the operating theatre and isolation wards. This was essential, she said, in order to establish 'the neatness and regularity' which had been so deficient.[75] After seven months in the hospital, the board declared that Coles's able and judicious direction of the nursing deserved the highest praise and had 'given unqualified satisfaction to the Committee and the Medical Staff'.[76] When the *Lancet* carried out a survey of night nursing in the London hospitals in 1871, its visitors were unimpressed with the night nurses, but described Coles as 'an active and intelligent person' and a good supervisor who worked gratis.[77] When she died unexpectedly in 1874, the board commented on her ability and energy and how greatly she had improved the moral tone of the hospital.[78]

In 1884 the BNA's generosity finally caught up with it. In the 1881–82 fiscal year, the BNA's revenue from hospital and private nursing was £1,274 6s. 0d., and its expenses £1,574 14s. 10d. The governors made up the deficit with subscriptions, donations and the sale of securities, but by 1884 realized the BNA was going bankrupt. They dismissed 13 women who were doing private nursing, leaving 30 nurses at the Royal Free and eight at the Hampstead Hospital. The BNA offered to transfer their organization and home to St Mary's Hospital if suitable terms could be arranged, but St Mary's was not interested.[79] On 30 June 1884 the BNA terminated its contract with the Royal Free and dissolved.[80]

The Royal Free Hospital then decided to establish its own nursing service. They asked Miss Carberry, who had succeeded Miss Coles in 1874, to remain as lady superintendent, and invited all of her staff who wished to stay on to do so. Only one or two nurses left. The hospital then brought the nurses' salaries into line with those of other hospitals. The new nursing service cost the hospital £1,014 2s. 1d. in its first year, compared to the BNA's cost of £715 18s. 10d. in fiscal year 1883.[81]

Like the two sisterhoods in their three hospitals, the BNA had greatly improved the nursing at the Royal Free, enabling its doctors to undertake more advanced practice. As it did the sisterhoods, religious ardour motivated the BNA board. Its most active board members were committed evangelical army officers. General Marshall supplied copies of tracts on prayer to be distributed to the patients, and

---

74    See, for example, RFH/WB, 11 August 1874.
75    RFH/WB, 16 June 1870; 14, 21, and 28 December 1871; 11 January 1873.
76    RFH/A6, p. 11.
77    *Lancet*, 11 November 1871, pp. 680–81.
78    RFH/WB, 17 September 1874.
79    SM/AD1/16, 28 March, 25 April 1884.
80    RFH/WB, 10 July 1884.
81    RFH/A8 (1884), p. 14; RFH/A/9 (1885), p. 13.

General Lawrence arranged for Miss Robinson to address the nurses, convalescent patients and their friends and families on the subject of temperance. Many of the nurses were already total abstainers. General Wilmot invited hospital board members to the BNA's annual prayer meeting.[82] These were all characteristic evangelical practices.[83] The army officers constantly pushed the hospital board to upgrade the working and living conditions and diet of the nurses.[84] In 1872, General Wilmot personally paid half the cost of improvements to the nurses' dormitory, and in 1874 the BNA fitted up, at its own cost, another room as a dormitory for extra nurses and probationers even though the hospital maintained the right to repossess the room if it needed it.[85] When they renegotiated the contract with the hospital in 1878, the BNA was paying for the nurses' food. Pointing out that their charges were lower than nursing costs in other hospitals, the BNA representatives told the board that they could no longer afford to supply the lady superintendent at their own cost, and suggested the hospital pay her £60.[86] As hospital nursing became more labour-intensive and sophisticated, it became more expensive, and small private charities became less able to subsidize it.

**The View from Outside**

The governors of the four hospitals using the central system were most enthusiastic about it, but how did those outside these hospitals evaluate it? From the beginning, external observers were impressed with the Sisters' nursing. In 1855, visitors commented on the 'happy looks' of the paid nurses.[87]

In 1858, ladies from a nurse training institution in Liverpool visited St John's House to study its rules and discipline; they were very impressed.[88] Florence Nightingale, a particularly shrewd observer, declared in 1863 that the best system of nursing was 'where nurses are of a religious order, and are under their own spiritual head; the institution being administered by a separate and secular governing body'[89] – precisely the sisterhood system. But Nightingale also identified the basic flaw in that system when she wrote in 1866 that there were not enough women willing to work as unpaid nursing Sisters to meet the rapidly increasing

[82]   RFH/WB, 22 February 1872, 3 April 1873, 14 December 1871, 25 February 1875.
[83]   Chadwick, *The Victorian Church*, vol. 1, pp. 440–43.
[84]   See, for example, RFH/WB, 14 December 1871; ibid., 11, 18 and 25 July 1872; ibid., 24 April, 14 May, 25 September, 6 November 1873.
[85]   RFH/WB, 28 July 1872, 18 June 1874.
[86]   RFH/WB, 7 March 1878.
[87]   LMA/H01/ST/SJ/A20/3, 10 October, 1855.
[88]   LMA/H01/ST/SJ/A20/4, 31 July 1857, 26 May 1858.
[89]   Florence Nightingale, *Notes on Hospitals* (3rd edn, London, 1863), pp. 181–2.

demand.[90] Nevertheless, St John's House continued to successfully train religious Sisters, so that there were 35 in 1883.[91]

The St John's House Sisters had only been at King's College Hospital some months when their dramatic improvements became apparent to the governors and doctors of the other teaching hospitals. The central system had a major impact at Guy's and St Thomas'. In August 1856, Mrs Turner, the wife of the treasurer at Guy's, came to St John's House to consult on improving patient care at Guy's.[92] Dr Steele, the administrator at Guy's, studied the central system,[93] and in April 1857 introduced a number of its measures. He employed charwomen to lighten the duties of the nurses, but to offset the cost, reduced the number of nurses. He also provided the nurses with full board and considered having them served their meals together with the sisters in a dining room as at King's. He decided against this because he did not have enough staff to cover the wards while half went off for their meals. However, Steele evinced no interest in the instruction which Jones thought so essential.[94]

In 1858, St Thomas' Hospital incorporated parts of the central system. The hospital reduced the number of sisters in its newly rebuilt North Wing, and as at King's College Hospital, employed a few ladies who each supervised several wards. St Thomas' gave these sisters and nurses full board; sisters and nurses ate together with a sister presiding, and all lived in the hospital at hospital expense. The nurses had formerly done all the cleaning; now the hospital hired a scrubber for each ward and also relieved the nurses of scrubbing the staircases.[95] These adaptations of the St John's House system were real improvements in the nurses' working and living conditions, but ignored the feature the Sisters thought most important: instruction. Even after the Nightingale School opened in 1860, Florence Nightingale believed there was no real teaching until Maria Machin became Home Sister in 1874.[96]

Word of the Sisters' success spread quickly throughout Europe. In 1857 the Grand Duke and Duchess of Hesse and delegations from the King of Prussia, Napoleon III and Czar Alexander II all visited King's College Hospital to study the Sisters' nursing arrangements. Florence Nightingale also visited the hospital.[97] Many other organizations and individuals, not the least of whom was Florence Nightingale, sought Jones's advice. Doctors and administrators at three London teaching hospitals, the Westminster, University College and St George's, were so

[90]   LMA/H01/ST/NC1/66/24.

[91]   See Chapter 9, p. XXX.

[92]   LMA/H01/ST/SJ/A20/3, 30 August 1856.

[93]   LMA/H09/GY/A164/1/1, p. 12.

[94]   LMA/H09/GY/A67/1, 5 August 1857.

[95]   LMA/H01/ST/A44/2 pp. 77–8; LMA/H01/ST/A50, 27 April 1858.

[96]   BL 47719, fols 122–3.

[97]   CSSJD, F.F. Cartwright, 'The Story of St John's House', *KCH Nurses' League Journal* (1959): p. 34.

impressed that they asked St John's House to take over their nursing. Jones refused St George's because Nightingale had warned her that the hospital was badly managed, and the other two hospitals because she did not have enough nurses.[98]

One well-informed observer of the St John's House achievements was Florence Lees. In January 1868, Jones and six of her eight Sisters withdrew from St John's House. Because the hospital's contract was with St John's House, the Sisters had to withdraw from King's College Hospital as well.[99] Two Sisters and the paid working-class nurses whom Jones had trained remained behind. While it was recruiting and training new Sisters, the St John's House council staffed the hospital with temporary sisters, of whom Florence Lees was one in early 1868. She had 'trained' at St Thomas' in 1866, but as an observer rather than a probationer.[100] Lees was very interested in the 'tone' of hospitals. The immorality in many of the old hospitals was notorious, she said. As well, probationers accepted fees from patients and appropriated their food and stimulants.[101] Hospital administrators shared Lees' concern with improving the tone of hospital life,[102] as we have seen at St George's, where the governors appreciated that the altercations between Cheeseley and Steel were very destructive of staff morale.

In contrast, the tone at King's College Hospital deeply impressed Lees. Lectures were given twice a week in the dispensary for sisters who cared to attend, while a senior physician gave lectures on simple pathology. There were seven new sisters, but the assistant nurses were the old St John's House-trained nurses. The excellent discipline of these nurses who had trained under Jones, Lees thought remarkable. She reported to Nightingale:

> I thought both wards and hospital in admirable order and well worked, partly owing to the kindness of the medical men and partly to the implicit obedience with which their orders were carried out. I have heard high praise of the general management from various sources both during the time I was there and since.[103]

## Diffusion of the Sisters' System

A look at the eight teaching hospitals which were not using the central system indicates that in 1856, St John's House was decades ahead of them in establishing an efficient nursing service. The achievement of St John's House as the leader in nineteenth-century nursing reform, however, has been obscured by the other

---

[98]   LMA/H01/ST/SJ/A20/3, 15 December 1855; LMA/H01/ST/SJ/A20/4, 25 May 1857; BL 47743 fols 50–51; BL 47744 fols 62–3.

[99]   See Chapter 9, pp. XXX–XXX.

[100]  LMA/H01/ST/NTS/C1/1, p. 6.

[101]  LMA/A/NFC/22/4, p. 10.

[102]  Helmstadter, 'A Real Tone': pp. 3–30.

[103]  BL 47756, fols 32–3.

hospitals appearing to have 'training schools' for nurses. In practice, these 'schools' amounted to improved accommodation and board, and not, as we would now expect, the provision of formal instruction.

In 1867 the Middlesex hired University College Hospital-trained Miss Catherine Martyr to establish what the hospital called a training school.[104] The following year, the governors began building a fine new nurses' home. It was to have a dining room, sitting room, laundry and bathroom. Cubicles with walls six feet high and a curtain at the end provided the bedrooms.[105] Martyr awarded certificates to the probationers after three years, but there is no evidence that she arranged any formal instruction.[106] Many hospitals awarded certificates to women who had worked a certain length of time without any formal training,[107] so this was not unusual. Martyr's successor, Miss Miriam Thorold, matron from 1870 to 1905, was also All Saints-trained. Thorold listed subjects, copied verbatim from the Nightingale Training School curriculum, which the probationers were supposed to learn, but there was no medical instruction and she herself gave no nursing classes.[108]

Harriet Coster, matron of St George's Hospital from 1872 to 1897, was a clinically experienced nurse, but not one of the new 'trained' nurses. She operated as an old-style matron. Perhaps in consequence, St George's was among the last of the teaching hospitals to introduce formalized training.[109] At the Westminster, the two Merryweather sisters, Mary and Elizabeth, established a school in 1874 when the governors rented a comfortable home in Queen Square for the probationers. The Merryweathers advertised themselves as Nightingale-trained nurses, but had spent only two months in 1862 observing at St Thomas' before taking on direction of the Liverpool Royal Infirmary's nursing institution. Miss Mary Merryweather said she held classes in the nurses' home on subjects such as anatomy and physiology, but there were no medical lectures and no evidence of systematic training. It was not until 1880, when Mary Jane Pyne, who trained at the Nightingale School and had been assistant superintendent at the Edinburgh Royal Infirmary, became lady superintendent, that real nursing instruction was introduced.[110]

---

[104]   C. Helmstadter, 'Building a New Nursing Service: Respectability and Efficiency in Victorian England', *Albion*, 35/4 (2003): pp. 602–4.

[105]   MH/MBG, 27 July 1866; MH/Minutes of Sub-committees, Nursing Committee 1867–1892, 22 March, 14–15 November 1867; *Lancet*, 18 July 1868, pp. 91–2; LMA/ H01/A/NFC/22/4, p. 21.

[106]   Helmstadter, 'Building a New Nursing Service', p. 605.

[107]   See, for example, LH/A17/3, 29 October, 3 December 1822; LMA/H09/GY/ ph8/1/5, 6 and 13.

[108]   LMA/A/NFC/22/4, p. 21.

[109]   S. Hawkins, *Nursing and Women's Labour in the Nineteenth Century: The Quest for Independence* (London, 2010), pp. 34, 176–7.

[110]   Humble and Hansell, *Westminster Hospital 1716–1966*, pp. 83–4; LMA/H02/WH/ A1/45, 8 December 1874; LMA/A/NFC/22/4, pp. 43–4.

At the other five hospitals, the training schools were directed by the old housekeeper matrons who were not nurses. The London started its school in 1873, awarding certificates to assistant nurses after three years of service. The probationers slept in their own home adjoining the hospital, but it had no dining or sitting rooms. There was no formal instruction until Miss Eva Lückes became matron in 1880.[111] Guy's introduced a school for lady probationers in the late 1870s. Dr Steele and the dispenser gave weekly lectures, but the lady probationers were not a success, and were discontinued.[112] It was not until after 1879, when St John's House-trained Margaret Burt became matron, that a real training school was established.[113] Bart's started its training school in 1877. Members of the medical staff gave the instruction, which consisted of eight medical and five surgical lectures a year as well as some instruction from the doctors on the wards. An effective training school at Guy's, as at St Thomas', only started when St Thomas'-trained Maria Machin became matron in 1879.[114]

Mrs Alicia Wright, matron of St Mary's from its opening in 1851 until 1876, did not even attempt to supervise, much less instruct the nurses. She was twice threatened with dismissal for inefficiency and failure to maintain discipline, but managed to hang on until she was 65 years old.[115] She was followed by Rachel Williams, who had trained at the Nightingale School. Williams reorganized the nursing, recruiting probationers to save money,[116] and setting up a small library and common room for the nurses. By 1883 she was giving weekly lectures on 'details of nursing', while the medical men gave lectures 'from time to time' on medical and surgical nursing. The doctors forced Williams to resign in 1885, and it was her successor, Miss Medill, who introduced a more thorough training.[117]

St Thomas' was a unique case: it had the Nightingale Training School from 1860, but until 1887, when Sarah Wardroper, matron since 1854, retired, it was another school directed by a woman who was not a nurse. After 1874 there was a carefully planned curriculum of lectures given during the day by the doctors, but the probationers often could not be spared from their ward work to attend. When they could attend, many were so tired they fell asleep. The Home Sister

[111]   Ibid., pp. 64–5; C. Daunton, *The London Hospital Illustrated: 250 Years* (London, 1990), p. 82.

[112]   LMA/H09/GY/225/2, p. 127; LMA/H09/GY/224/3, pp. 6–8.

[113]   H.C. Cameron, *Mr. Guy's Hospital 1726–1948* (London, 1954), p. 203.

[114]   SB/MC/1/1, 1 April, 22 July 1876; SBH, Sister Casualty, 'A Reformation', *St. Bartholomew's League News* (May 1902); SBH/Ha1/24, 5 and 12 December 1878; SBH/Ha3/13, 14 March 1880.

[115]   LMA/A/NFC/22/4, p. 57; E.A. Heaman, *St Mary's: The History of a London Teaching Hospital* (Montreal, 2003), p. 31.

[116]   Probationers were generally paid less than half as much as the assistant nurses whom they replaced.

[117]   SM/AD1/14, 3 and 10 November 1876, 15 March 1878; SM/AD/13/3, 5 November 1883; Heaman, *St Mary's*, pp. 114–15.

gave lectures in the nurses' home in the evening after work, but many probationers snored through them, as Nightingale put it, for the same reason.[118] Nightingale conferred extensively with Jones in the early 1860s, and thus St John's House had considerable influence on the ideals of the school, though much less in practice. Indeed, Jones became one of Nightingale's closest friends and her chief mentor when she was drawing up the rules for her school. Jones strongly recommended that the matron have the authority to engage and dismiss both probationers and the nurses whom the hospital paid.[119] Unlike most matrons, the matron at St Thomas' had always had this power. She retained it under the contract with the Nightingale Fund Council, something which, as Wardroper became increasingly senile,[120] Nightingale was later to regret.[121]

**Conclusion**

Nightingale and Jones had both separately come to the conclusion that proper training for nurses could only be achieved with clinical experience in a teaching hospital, but it was Jones who convinced Nightingale that the working-class nurses had to be treated with more kindness and have better working conditions. For example, Jones thought the seven hours' sleep allowed the night nurses inadequate; she recommended eight. She allowed her probationers a candle on nights, not just the gas turned down to its lowest flame, and she encouraged them to knit on duty. 'It is dreary work indeed,' she explained, 'to watch in a large ward with only the glimmering of the gas turned down very low.' Nightingale asked Jones to comment on the Monthly Register she had drawn up. This was the famous character sheet, based on Kaiserswerth practice, which the sisters were supposed to complete weekly and the matron monthly, assessing each probationer's personal characteristics and nursing skills. Jones tactfully commented that it was very carefully designed, but pointed out it was unlikely to be properly implemented because it required so much time to fill out accurately.[122]

Jones had many reservations about the St Thomas's contract. She found the governors' attitude disturbing. In her view, they should aim to make nursing a respectable and desirable employment. Rather than trying to improve the nursing, the governors seemed more interested in making the school a paying business for the hospital. She thought they were overcharging the Nightingale Fund, and found it distressing that so wealthy a hospital was not more liberal. Furthermore, the one-

---

[118] See, for example, LMA/H01/ST/NTS/Y17/2; BL 47719 fol. 84; BL 47745, fols 45–6.
[119] BL 47743, fol. 13.
[120] BL 47738, fols 116–17, 350–52, 359–60; BL 47740, fols 39–41.
[121] Golding, *An Historical Account*, p. 204; LMA/H01/ST/A6/12, 10 April 1860.
[122] BL 47743, fols 28–9, 35–8; L. McDonald (ed.), *Florence Nightingale on Women, Medicine, Midwifery and Prostitution* (Waterloo, ON, 2005), pp. 51–2.

year contract they offered gave too little time to tell whether such an experiment would succeed, but on the other hand, Jones told Nightingale, St Thomas' offered no inducement to the Nightingale Fund to place themselves in their hands for a longer period.[123]

The two reforming matrons the Sisters trained – Margaret Burt, who introduced the new nursing at Guy's, and Sister Elizabeth, the first All Saints Sister-in-Charge at University College Hospital – provide another illustration of the leadership of St John's House in early nursing reform. As it did Nightingale, St John's House's also profoundly influenced other influential nursing leaders. In the 1860s, Nightingale insisted that future lady superintendents trained at St Thomas' also take some training at King's College Hospital. Among these ladies were Lucy Osburn, who was sent to Australia to found Nightingale nursing there, and Emmy Rappe, the Swedish nursing reformer.[124] At Nightingale's request, Jane Shaw Stewart, the unsuccessful first lady superintendent in a military hospital, had an extended stay with Jones. Unlike Nightingale, Jones correctly judged her failings, saying she was 'greatly mistaken on sundry points', but impossible to straighten out, and showed a 'dogged persistence in misapprehending and misrepresenting all one could say or do.'[125]

*Personal versus Professional Lives*

Jones had always had High Church tendencies. As she became more successful and more heavily burdened with hospital work, she expressed these leanings more overtly. In 1860, with the exception of Mrs Hodson, who was staunchly Low Church, she began calling the Sisters, in High Church style, Sister Bessie or Sister Louisa, rather than Miss Wallis or Miss Simcox.[126] In June 1865 the Sisters convinced their council to transfer the duties of secretary and treasurer from the Rev. Henry Giraud, the master, to Jones, making his sole function that of chaplain. Jones then took the distinctly High Church title of Mother Superior. The Sisters began avoiding the services which Giraud held, going instead to St Alban's, Holborn, the most notorious of the ritualistic churches.[127] Just as Jones and her Sisters were becoming more open about their ritualism[128] the reaction against the

---

[123]   BL 47743, fols 9–10, 14–15.

[124]   Godden, *Lucy Osburn*, pp. 62–4, 69–70; E. Rappe, *'God Bless You My Dear Miss Nightingale': Letters from Emily Carolina Rappe to Florence Nightingale 1867–1870* (Stockholm, 1977), pp. 24–5.

[125]   BL 47743, fols 98, 101.

[126]   LMA/H01/ST/SJ/A20/5, 16 July, 7 August 1860.

[127]   LPA, Tait Papers, vol. 149, fol. 241 (this folio is a booklet), pp. 6–7; LMA/H01/ST/SJ/A20/5, 14 July, 7 August 1860; SJ/A35/1, Letter of 19 September 1866, Letter of Henry Giraud to Bishop of London's Chaplain [1866], Letter in response, 6 October 1866.

[128]   Ritualism was a High Church movement which emphasized ancient ritual and elaborate vestments and trappings. Chadwick, *The Victorian Church*, vol. 2, pp. 310–11.

High Church movement, and sisterhoods in particular, reached its zenith. Fears that immoral practices resulting from celibacy, the secrecy of the confessional and stories of young women confined in convents against their will had led to unsuccessful efforts to establish inspection of convents in the 1850s. In the 1860s these anxieties resurfaced more powerfully, reaching a peak in 1864–65, when, in an effort to prevent 'Romanizing' the Established Church, a group of churchmen formed the Church Association, an organization devoted to resisting ritualism. They circulated floods of pamphlets attacking sisterhoods, which deeply wounded Jones.[129]

In this intensely inflamed atmosphere, matters came to a head at St John's House. Blomfield had resigned at the end of 1856; the new Bishop of London was Archibald Campbell Tait. Essentially a pragmatist, Tait was personally unsympathetic to High Church practices and discouraged ritualism. At the same time he recognized that the Church needed all the zeal it could find, and was prepared to support sisterhoods as long as they did not have life-long vows or practise frequent private confession.[130] Unfortunately for the Sisters, Tait did not have the same interest in nursing as Blomfield. When Jones sent her resignation to Tait as President of the St John's House Council, he did not even know how she was associated with St John's House.[131]

The Sisters wished to replace the Low Church Giraud with a High Church chaplain, W.W. Labarte, who would administer vows and hear confession – the very two things Tait would not tolerate.[132] Jones tried to convince Tait that although oaths, or vows, were illegal in the Anglican Church, a Sister's vow was not an oath but an act of private devotion. She wrote to Tait, speaking apologetically of her personal experience. 'I am an old woman now,' she said (she was 54), 'and I have seen this longing for the Religious life spreading widely and deeply among the daughters of our beloved Church.' She then went on to explain that for her, a vow brought strength and comfort. 'My own vow was many years ago, quite irrespective of St John's House,' she told Tait. She did not even know it existed then, but amidst many trials, sorrows and disappointments, and much arduous work, that personal vow had given her the strength to persevere. Tait was wrong in thinking that she forced compulsory confession on her Sisters; she had always said compulsory confession was an abuse.[133] The fact that she worked so well with Mrs Hodson indicates that Jones was being honest.

Tait was not sympathetic. 'You must be ready,' he wrote to Jones:

---

[129]   Arnstein, *Protestant vs. Catholic in Mid-Victorian England*, pp. 3–6, 44–8, 62–73; Chadwick, *The Victorian Church*, vol. 2, pp. 319–21; LMA/H01/ST/ NC1/66/25.

[130]   P.T. Marsh, 'Tait, Archibald Campbell (1811–82)', *Oxford Dictionary of National Biography*, <www.oxforddnb.com/view/article/26917> (accessed 10 July 2011).

[131]   BL 45752, fol. 252.

[132]   LPA, Tait Papers, vol. 148 fols 199–200, 204–5, 208–9.

[133]   Ibid., vol. 148, fols 211–12, 214–15.

to sacrifice your own individual tastes and wishes when those placed over you in the Lord ... advise that you should make the best of the circumstances in which you find yourselves and work steadily in spite of discouragements considering the great opportunities of Christian usefulness which are opened up to you in the sphere to which God's providence has called you.[134]

It was not a response which women who had sacrificed so much of their individual tastes and wishes to build an innovative nursing service would appreciate. In October 1867 the Sisters informed the bishop they were severing their connection with the St John's House Council.[135] 'We must demand the right to regulate our own inner life,' Jones told Tait.[136] Jones, six Sisters and a Probationary Sister resigned, and in January 1868 established their own independent sisterhood, the Sisterhood of St Mary and St John. The new sisterhood undertook district nursing, and eventually established a chronic care hospital,[137] which is still flourishing.

King's College Hospital desperately wanted to keep the Sisters, and asked Nightingale to intervene. Nightingale urged Jones to compromise. 'You must know how extremely anxious they are to retain the sisterhood,' she wrote Jones – in fact, so anxious that she thought Jones could dictate the terms.[138] Jones and her Sisters, however, had made their decision. The hospital governors deeply regretted their departure. It was impossible, they wrote, to express their 'deep sense of grateful obligation to the Sisters for the way in which they had performed their self-imposed duty' for 12 years. Jones replied that 'in the midst of all the pain involved' in separating from St John's House, leaving the hospital was one of the keenest. 'We shall retain a loving remembrance of our twelve years sojourn in King's College Hospital,' she declared.[139] The *British Medical Journal* summarized the medical viewpoint:

All who know what a great work these ladies have long been engaged in, and what an excellent staff of nurses they have trained for private patients, as well as for the wards of King's College Hospital, and lately for those of Charing Cross Hospital, will lament that the success and continuance of such a work should be threatened by a question of religious discipline.[140]

The aged Mrs Hodson had previously resigned because of ill health. The council now recalled her as lady superintendent and successfully recruited more Sisters

---

[134] Ibid., vol. 145, fols 361–2.
[135] Ibid., vol. 148, fols 216–17.
[136] Cited in Moore, *A Zeal for Responsibility*, p. 9. Since Moore wrote her book, this volume of the St John's House council minutes has become too fragile to be consulted.
[137] Ibid., p. 10.
[138] LMA/H01/ST/NC1/67/9.
[139] KH/CM/M7, 16 and 30 January 1868.
[140] *BMJ*, 11 January 1868, p. 33.

with Low Church leanings. In 1870 the council appointed Sister Caroline Lloyd Superior. Lloyd was well liked, and proved both able[141] and more willing to compromise than Jones. Emma Durham, who began training at King's College Hospital in 1872, reported going on nights in the traditional manner, after only five hours of rest from her day shift, and doing as much washing up as did the Nightingale probationers. She remembered blisters on her feet from walking up and down the ward, and on her hands from wringing out hot flannels for fomentations, but she also recorded that the probationers had an hour lecture-demonstration from the Sister or senior nurse every day after tea.[142] The sisterhood continued to nurse King's College Hospital successfully until 1883, when another struggle with the council over the autonomy of the sisterhood led all 35 Sisters to resign.[143]

*The Advantages and Disadvantages of Sisterhood Nursing*

The contemporary medical press accepted the Sisters as the leaders in modern nursing as enthusiastically as did the Sisters' hospitals boards. 'The nursing by ladies is the very best nursing that England has ever seen,' the *Lancet* declared in 1866. Sisterhood nursing embodied 'intelligence, keenest sympathy and refinement'.[144] 'The objections urged, and what is more unfortunate, practically adopted against sisterhoods as nurses into certain medical institutions,' the *British Medical Journal* (*BMJ*) stated:

> seems to us very regrettable, as well as ill-founded. Everyone admits the difficulty at this time of obtaining efficient, and above all educated nurses; and the difficulty does not seem likely to diminish, the demand for a fitting supply of attendants on the sick being continually on the increase.

It was sad that sisterhoods were rejected 'on the ground of their holding certain sectional views' when it had never been shown that they had done any proselytizing. In any case, the *BMJ* concluded, 'better too much religion than none at all'.[145] The *Medical Press and Circular* noted that Dr Steevens' Hospital in Dublin was introducing a secular lady superintendent to train probationers. 'This nursing system on an "unsectarian basis" looks very well,' the editor asserted,

---

[141]    KH/CM/M7, 9 January 1868; Moore, *A Zeal for Responsibility*, pp. 10, 12.

[142]    E.D., *Recollections of a Nurse* (London, 1889), p. 2; F.F. Cartwright, 'Nightingales and Eagles' (unpublished manuscript), pp. 196–9, 203. Cartwright was a historian of medicine, and this was his last work. He had access to another, fuller edition of *Recollections*, published by Macmillan in 1892 which is not in the British Library. We are indebted to Professor Lynn McDonald for a copy of Cartwright's manuscript.

[143]    Moore, *A Zeal for Responsibility*, pp. 11–39, 101–68.

[144]    *Lancet*, 6 September 1866, p. 271.

[145]    *BMJ*, 11 August 1866, p. 163; See also *BMJ*, 28 April, 5 May 1866, pp. 445, 476.

'but in London it is found that the sisterhood plan, such as that at King's College Hospital, works much better.'[146]

In 1868 the *Lancet* commented on the enormous difference between hospitals like St Bartholomew's which used the old nursing system, and those like King's College and University College Hospitals which employed ladies to superintend their nurses.[147] As was often the case, the writer did not mention that these ladies were religious Sisters. Like the lay hospital governors at Charing Cross, many doctors seemed to feel the superior social status of the Sisters was a more important factor in their success than their religious and educational commitment. It was also generally assumed in the 1860s that any improved nursing was based on the sisterhood system. For example, the *BMJ* reported in April 1866 that in Bristol, Bath and Liverpool there were successful schools for nurses based on the St John's House system.[148] Although there were lady superintendents and somewhat improved nursing at these hospitals, Sister Mary Jones would never have agreed that their nursing was based on the sisterhood system.

In 1874 the *BMJ* set up a commission to study nursing systems in the London teaching hospitals. Like Golding in 1819, the commissioners thought that nursing was 'a constant source of trouble and anxiety' to hospital administrators, demonstrated by the many years and experiments spent trying to remedy it. Golding had thought it was simply a question of finding 'proper persons'; some 50 years later, the *BMJ* pronounced it a far more complex matter.[149] The sisterhoods had solved the problem of respectability and efficiency, the *BMJ* explained, but the solution brought many new problems. It saw the two most important problems as first, that it was generally and erroneously believed 'lady nursing' was more expensive, and second, the independent authority, or what came to be called the *imperium in imperio*,[150] which the Sisters' contracts created inside their hospitals.[151] A third major problem, which the *BMJ* did not take in but which Florence Nightingale recognized, was the insufficient number of educated women willing to enter nursing as unpaid religious Sisters.[152]

The *BMJ* commissioners named four hospitals as having improved systems of nursing: the three nursed by the sisterhoods and St Thomas'. Why they omitted the Royal Free is not explained – possibly because it was just establishing its medical school in 1874. The commissioners had included St Thomas', they explained, because it had a lady superintendent and lady sisters, but they thought it differed from the other three hospitals in every other respect, so they did not include it

---

146  *Medical Press and Circular*, 15 August 1866, p. 181.
147  *Lancet*, 6 November 1869, p. 650.
148  *BMJ*, 21 April 1866, pp. 419–20.
149  *BMJ*, 28 February 1874, p. 285.
150  'Empire within an empire'.
151  *BMJ*, 14 March 1874, p. 357.
152  LMA/H01/ST/NC1/66/25.

in the rest of their discussion.[153] In fact, despite the Nightingale Fund Council's advertising, few accorded Sarah Wardroper the status of a lady, and there were few lady sisters at St Thomas' in 1874.

The commissioners saw three advantages to sisterhood nursing. First, patients and nurses more readily obeyed a lady; second, her presence checked 'rough play and coarse joking', and third, she was likely to be more conscientious because she was working out of commitment rather than for the money. The disadvantages were that first, ladies were not used to taking orders, so to be successful, they had to have either 'unusual tact, judgment and general power of management', or there must be the strong *esprit de corps* for which the sisterhoods were noted and which the *BMJ* considered the primary cause of their success. After carefully weighing the advantages and disadvantages of sisterhood nursing, the commissioners concluded that it was the best system.[154] It was not, however, to be the system of the future.

---

[153]   *BMJ*, 4 April 1874, p. 462.
[154]   *BMJ*, 14 March, 4 April 1874, pp. 357 and 462.

# Chapter 9
# The Demise of Sisterhood Nursing
# and the Central System

Sisterhood nursing had revolutionized hospital nursing services, and in the 1860s and 1870s was much in demand. By 1880, St John's House was turning out large numbers of trained nurses. Between 1870 and 1880, the Sisters trained 850 nurses.[1] In comparison, in the same decade the Nightingale School accepted 372 women, of whom only 242 completed their training.[2] Other teaching hospitals incorporated less expensive aspects of the Sisters' system, but they paid little attention to the instruction in nursing skills and knowledge which was such an important part of the Sisters' system.[3] In 1872 alone, the St John's House Sisters, because of insufficient personnel, turned down requests to take over the nursing at 11 different hospitals, including Addenbrooke's in Cambridge and a Birmingham hospital.[4] In 1888, the All Saints Sisters turned down a request to nurse a hospital in Hong Kong for the same reason. As well as University College Hospital, they were then nursing the Metropolitan Hospital in London, three hospitals in Bombay and one in South Africa.[5]

Individual St John-trained nurses also helped disseminate the Sisters' system. Mary Weedon, who nursed at Charing Cross from 1878 to 1881, emigrated to Australia and established a similar training system at Brisbane Hospital when she was appointed matron there in 1886. It was the first comprehensive training programme in general nursing for laity in the colony of Queensland.[6] Grace Neill, a nursing reformer in New Zealand largely responsible for what is reputed to be the first national Act to register nurses, is another eminent nurse assumed to have been trained 'to Florence Nightingale's ideals'. In fact, she trained at St John's during 1873–76 and had no direct association with the Nightingale School at

[1]   CSSJD, Annual Report 1880.

[2]   L. McDonald (ed.), *Florence Nightingale: The Nightingale School* (Waterloo, ON, 2009), p. 38. Note that McDonald appears to include nurses, such as Maria Machin and Lucy Osburn, who were ill during their training, and so trained for far less than the year nominally required.

[3]   Williams, 'Religion, Respectability and the Origins of the Modern Nurse', p. 248.

[4]   LMA/H01/ST/SJ/Y9.

[5]   Mumm, *Stolen Daughters, Virgin Mothers*, p. 114.

[6]   H. Gregory, *A Tradition of Care: A History of Nursing at the Royal Brisbane Hospital* (Brisbane: Boolarong Publications, 1988), pp. 21–3.

St Thomas'.[7] Similarly, it was an All Saints Sister, Sister Helen Bowden, who in 1873 established the first training school in the United States at Bellevue Hospital in New York. Bowden had trained with the All Saints Sisters, was part of their first-class team in the Franco–Prussian War,[8] and never had anything to do with Nightingale or the Nightingale Training School. Regardless, the hospital tends to be silent about its All Saints connection, while promoting its school as, to take one typical phrasing, 'The nation's first nursing school based on Florence Nightingale's principles'.[9] A member of an Anglican sisterhood, Henrietta Stockdale, was responsible for the first nurse training school in Southern Africa. She trained with the Clewer Sisters and later under the All Saints' Sisters: she at least has largely escaped the assumption that she was associated with Nightingale.[10]

Yet despite their enormous success, the two nursing sisterhoods and the British Nursing Association were gone from the London teaching hospitals by 1900: St John's House in 1883, the BNA in 1884, and the All Saints Sisters in 1899. Why? Religious objections to sisterhoods and issues of gender and power within the hospital organization all played major roles in the demise of the central system. The vastly improved nursing and the ability to provide adequate numbers of reliable nurses which these organizations provided enabled the doctors to do a great deal more work, much of which was very costly to the hospital. In the case of the sisterhoods this was a key factor, for most people thought the Sisters, rather than the increased medical activity, caused the higher expenditures. As increasing numbers of nurses were required, both the All Saints Sisters and the BNA found themselves less and less able to continue subsidizing their hospitals at the rate at which they had started in 1862 and 1870.

**The Cost of the Central System of Nursing**

The insistence on reasonable staffing and living conditions as well as training, which itself necessitated heavier staffing, did seem to result in increased nursing costs.[11] However, the sisterhoods and the BNA, not the hospitals, bore much of the additional costs. In the 1850s and 1860s, the Sisters had the only trained and efficient nursing services in London. In the 1870s, the BNA added a fourth hospital. The

---

[7]    M. Tennant, 'Neill, Elizabeth Grace 1846–1926'. *Dictionary of New Zealand Biography*, <http://www.teara.govt.nz/en/biographies/2n5/1> (accessed 10 July 2011). We thank Marilyn Gendek for the reminder about Neill and Stockdale (see below).

[8]    ASA, Mother Foundress Box, Diary of Franco-Prussian War, pp. 1, 15, 21–2.

[9]    <http://medicine.med.nyu.edu/about-us/nyu-hospitals-and-affiliates/bellevue-hospital-center> (accessed 10 July 2011).

[10]    W.M. Buss and V. Buss, *The Lure of the Stone: The Story of Henrietta Stockdale* (Cape Town, H. Timmins, 1976).

[11]    See, for example, J.G. Wilkinson, *Hospital Relief and the Cost of its Administration in the Metropolis* (London, 1868), pp. 6–7.

other seven hospitals, which had to pay their nurses' costs themselves, had not yet found a way to fund the better working and living conditions which the sisterhoods and the BNA offered and subsidized and which the Nightingale Fund paid for at the twelfth hospital, St Thomas'.

This situation started to change in the 1870s. The other hospitals began establishing what they called nursing schools, although usually, as we have seen, these 'schools' differed only from the old nursing services in that they offered better room and board for the probationers. The new schools were also completely under the hospitals' control, hence hospital administrators were able to enforce economies and lower nurse-to-patient ratios which the Sisters and the BNA, with the greater autonomy their contracts conferred, refused to accept. Still, even if working conditions remained as harsh as ever, more respectable living conditions were a big drawing card for what administrators at these eight hospitals called 'a better class of woman'.

'With the improvement in therapeutics the function of the nurse has risen in importance,' the *Lancet* announced in 1868,[12] but just when nurses were becoming recognized as an important component in hospital practice, hospital revenues were diminishing. The successes of the new medicine caused budgetary crises in a number of the teaching hospitals. The steadily growing nursing staffs which the new therapeutics required were one cause,[13] while the agricultural depression of 1873–96 resulted in a dramatic fall in the hospitals' revenues. In fiscal year 1825, St Bartholomew's, the richest of the 12 hospitals, spent £5,023 less than its income of £39,894 and was able to invest the surplus.[14] By 1880, Bart's was borrowing money to meet its running expenses and had to sell £53,061 of its assets to meet its annual costs of £108,879.[15] Most of the teaching hospitals had always been under-funded, and their administrators, as at King's College Hospital in 1843 and University College Hospital in 1851 when Lister personally solicited donations to pay for more night nurses, saw nursing as the best place to economize. By the 1890s, the hospital-controlled training schools offered viable, less expensive alternatives to the central system.

The four hospitals that the BNA and two sisterhoods nursed so successfully were among the least well endowed. When other hospitals found cheaper ways of providing respectable and better-disciplined nurses, the financially pinched boards at King's College and University College Hospitals began objecting to the Sisters' costs. In 1874, the King's governors complained that their nursing costs and nurse-to-patient ratio was the highest of the eight teaching hospitals they had consulted. The Sisters attributed their heavier staffing to the spaciousness and configuration

---

[12]   *Lancet*, 14 March 1868, p. 353.

[13]   Smith, *The People's Health*, pp. 278–84.

[14]   SBH/HB21/4.

[15]   SBH/HB22/31. Prices remained steady during 1825–80, with inflation averaging -0.4 per cent per year; <http://www.bankofengland.co.uk/education/inflation/calculator/flash/index.htm> (accessed 10 July 2011).

of the wards in their new state-of-the-art hospital, the unusually large number of beds which were kept constantly occupied, and the exceptionally large number of critically ill patients and major surgical procedures. All these factors, they said, made King's College Hospital pre-eminent, but they also made its nursing more costly as they required a larger and better-trained nursing staff.[16] The Sisters also contested the governors' figures. Their own calculations showed the cost per nurse per year in the London teaching hospitals ranged from £40 11s. 9d. at the London to £61 16s. 0d. at the Westminster, with King's in the middle at £51 7s. 0d.[17]

The University College Hospital governors similarly suspected the All Saints Sisters of overstaffing. As at St John's House, beginning with their first contract the Sisters lost money, and the hospital recognized this. In January 1861, just three months after Sister Elizabeth took charge of two wards, Mother Harriet Brownlow Byron asked for more night nurses in these wards. She said she might have to withdraw her Sisters because nursing the two wards was so expensive. The committee extended the contract six months while it considered the matter, and in the meantime took on the expense of additional porters to relieve the nurses of carrying provisions and stores up to the wards.[18] In 1878, the hospital was paying the Sisters £1,638 a year when the Sisters' costs were £2,175 14s. 0d. The governors did not think the Sisters were overpaying in any area; on the contrary, they were concerned that they were not paying the older, experienced nurses enough to keep them from leaving. The hospital agreed to pay £182 more, £1,820 a year, leaving the Sisters to absorb an annual deficit of £233.[19]

In 1879, the hospital enlarged its building and reopened with a larger nursing staff of 53.[20] Two years later, the Sisters added a nurse and two probationers in the children's erysipelas and infectious wards. The governors asked the Medical Committee if the three additional nurses were really necessary. The doctors replied that the heavy nursing in those wards made the extra nurses essential.[21] By 1888, exclusive of the unpaid Sisters, there were 70 nurses and servants.[22] When in 1889, because of the increased workload, the Sisters asked the hospital to pay for more nurses, the governors replied that they could not afford more. The resident medical officer and Dr Barlow both attested that Sister Cecilia,[23] the Sister Superior (sometimes called Sister-in-Charge after 1882), could not manage with

---

[16]  LMA/H01/ST/SJ/A39/13, pp. iii–vi, 22–3.

[17]  LMA/H01/ST/SJ/A39/11.

[18]  UCH/A1/2/2, 15 January, 13 February, 24 April, 8 May, 17 and 31 July 1861.

[19]  UCH/A1/2/4, 4 and 18 December 1878.

[20]  ASA, UCH Box, unsigned Note, [1897]; UCH/A1/2/4, 9 June 1879.

[21]  UCH/A1/1/3, 16 February, 16 March 1881.

[22]  ASA, UCH Box, unsigned Note, [1897].

[23]  Records of the surnames for most of the All Saints Sisters have not survived, so, for consistency, we use their religious names.

fewer nurses.[24] In an effort to increase revenue in 1889, Sister Cecilia accepted seven probationers from other hospitals which paid her to train them.[25]

When in 1893 the governors established a committee to consider the high nurse-to-patient ratio, the Medical Committee informed them:

> Although the proportion of nurses to occupied beds is greater than at any other London hospital of corresponding size, your committee is not prepared to say that the number of nurses is excessive regard being had to the large number of serious cases admitted to the ward and the gradual increase in the proportion of such cases during the last ten to fifteen years.[26]

In July 1896, the governors decided the hospital was in such critical financial condition that they absolutely had to decrease the number of nurses. They again believed their nursing costs were the highest of comparable hospitals: 1 nurse to 2½ beds as compared to the other hospitals which ranged from 1:3¼ to 1:3⅞. The Medical Committee again insisted it was not possible to reduce the number of nurses.[27]

The comparisons with other hospitals were not entirely fair, as the Sisters and doctors pointed out, for those hospitals operated with 15–20 per cent of beds closed or empty, either kept for emergency cases or closed for lack of funds,[28] University College, King's College and the London Hospitals being exceptions. Despite the governors' desperate attempts to reduce the number of nurses, in 1897–98 they approved the addition of three more nurses – a Sister, a trained nurse and a probationer for the operating room[29] – another indication of the hospital's heavy surgical programme. In fact, the All Saints Sisters did not overstaff: in each instance, when the governors tried to cut back on the number of nurses, the doctors insisted the nurses were absolutely necessary.

Like the British Nursing Association, both sisterhoods thought of their hospital work as Christian philanthropy, and did not originally think of the hospital's underpayment as a financial loss. Rather, they saw it as a charitable contribution the sisterhoods were making to the sick poor. Hence, All Saints and St John's House had always been willing to undertake hospital nursing at a financial cost to themselves. By October 1897, however, Sister Cecilia wrote to the Mother Superior that the deficit had reached £1,250[30] – an amount which even All Saints, one of the wealthiest sisterhoods, could not afford. The Sisters had only £25 in the

24    ASA, UCH Box, *Nurses' League Magazine*, 13/15 (1973): p. 9.
25    UCH/A1/2/6, 6 November 1889.
26    UCH/A1/2/7, 15 March 1893.
27    UCH/A1/2/8, 22 July 1896; UCH/A1/5/2, 1 and 13 July 1896.
28    *PP* (1890), vol. 16, pp. 195–8.
29    UCH/A1/2/8, 8 December 1897, 20 April 1898.
30    [Sister Cecilia] to Gentlemen, [1897]. The hospital calculated the deficit at £1284 15s. 3d.; ASA, UCH Box, First Report of Special Committee, 22 December 1897.

bank and £108 16s. 6d. in accounts receivable, and the Nurses' Home from which their private nursing service operated was £350 in debt.[31] Sister Cecilia thought quite accurately that the deficit was a result of underpayment by the hospital, and believed less correctly that the Hospital Committee was beginning to realize that it must help the sisterhood with what was really its own deficit. She asked if in the mean time the sisterhood could lend her £400 to cover the debt at the Nurses' Home. Then she hoped that with the appeal which the Sisters were launching and the earnings of the private nurses, they could balance their accounts.[32]

As had the Sisters at St John's House, the All Saints Sisters made generous gifts to the hospital. In 1890, Sister Cecilia received a £970 legacy from her uncle which she gave to the hospital to clear its deficit. In 1892, the sisterhood donated £370 for the Chapel Fund and Nurses' Home. The Sisters also lent the hospital money: in 1885, £500 which the hospital paid off in 1890, and in 1893 another £500 of which £400 was still owing in 1897.[33] Sister Agnes Mary, Acting Sister-in-Charge from January 1898 when Sister Cecilia went on sick leave,[34] compared the All Saints costs with those of the nursing in other hospitals. Like the doctors in 1893, she thought it was comparing apples and oranges because the University College Hospital had such a large, active and enterprising medical school and did more major surgery than other hospitals. The introduction of aseptic technique in the later 1890s added to the burden. 'The work', Sister Agnes Mary explained, 'has increased enormously in the scientific direction.' All Saints did maintain a large nursing staff, but she did not see how they could manage with fewer nurses. Her figures gave an even lower nurse-to-patient ratio than those of the committee.[35] She compared four teaching hospitals operating with secular nursing systems to University College Hospital. The ratio of nurse to beds was: 1:4.4 at the Royal Infirmary Edinburgh; 1:3 at the Middlesex; 1:2.6 at Charing Cross; 1:2.3 at King's College; and 1:2.1 at University College. She pointed out that the Sisters did not employ ward maids as did most hospitals, which meant they needed more assistant nurses for the cleaning. Also, Sister Agnes Mary indicated, the hospital served a larger number of patients, 3,055 annually compared to 2,468 at King's, a hospital of similar size but with a secular nursing service since 1883.[36]

Sister Cecilia submitted all of these figures to the committee, regretting that she had not done this many years earlier because the hospital's payments for the nursing had not covered the costs since she had been in charge (in fact, they never

---

[31]    ASA, UCH Box, [Sister Cecilia] to Mother Superior, 27 October 1897.

[32]    Ibid.

[33]    ASA, UCH Box, 'Statement of Loans Gifts', [1897].

[34]    UCH/A1/2/8, 5 and 19 January 1898.

[35]    This ratio does not refer to the patient load of an individual nurse as it normally does today, but to the number of nurses compared to the number of patients or, more usually, beds in the hospital.

[36]    ASA, UCH Box, Statement of loans and gifts, [1897], no signature; Sister Agnes Mary to Mother Superior, 24 June 1897; 'Proportion of Nurses to Patients'.

had). The contract under which they were operating in 1897 had been signed in 1885, when there were 50 nurses. In 1897, there were over 100 on staff and the hospital was paying the Sisters the same £192 5s. 0d. a month when their costs were £266 5s. 4d.[37] In addition to the wages of the larger staff, Sister Cecilia explained, there were other reasons for the sisterhood's increased costs: a newly appointed nurse to keep order in the Out-Patient Department, and two new district nurses, the expense of the room, board and laundry for the additional nurses, an extra servant for the Nurses' Home, outdoor uniforms, and better-quality food because their nurses now came from a better class. Also, Sister Cecilia did not insist on payments from paying probationers who were not well off.[38] Over the four years 1894–97 she had collected £2,884 13s. 10d., or 92 per cent of the £3,148 8s. which they owed. Even so, the cost of the 107 Sisters, nurses and servants on Sister Cecilia's staff was 10s. 7d. per head per week, while the cost at King's was 13s. 11d.[39] This lower cost, of course, was caused in part because the religious Sisters worked without pay. Dr Steele, the highly competent, thrifty professional administrator at Guy's, thought in 1869 that University College Hospital was getting a real bargain with the Sisters' nursing.[40] Sister Cecilia had always hoped that the pupils' fees would make up the deficit, but she now asked the hospital to increase its monthly payment from £192 5s. 0d. to £225 a month. The Sisters were prepared to absorb a cost of over £41 a month, almost £500 annually, when the hospital owed them £400.

Most of the teaching hospitals sent some of their trained or partially trained nurses to families for private nursing. The families paid the hospital considerably more – at least twice as much and more in the case of fever patients – than the hospital paid the nurses for their private work, thus generating a profit for the hospital,[41] but Sister Cecilia had co-mingled the monies for the private and hospital nursing in one bank account. If the private nurses had a good year, she used the surplus to help pay the hospital nurses' deficit and vice-versa.[42] The governors estimated that she had used approximately £500 for the hospital nursing service which should have gone into their coffers. The governors demanded that the Sisters pay them £784 15s. 3d. to cover the debts incurred up to 31 December 1897, and that they make up any income received from private nursing in 1898 which has been used to pay those debts.[43] The hospital did agree to pay for the room and

[37] Ibid., [Sister Cecilia] to Gentlemen, [1897].

[38] All the hospitals had 'lady probationers': women who paid for their training, usually a guinea a week, although sometimes less.

[39] ASA, UCH Box, First Report of the Special Committee to consider the costs of the nursing and servants, 22 December 1897.

[40] J.C. Steele, 'Statistical Account of the Patients Treated in Guy's Hospital', *Guy's Hospital Reports*, 3rd Series, vol. 16 (London, 1871), pp. 548–9.

[41] Abel-Smith, *A History of the Nursing Profession*, pp. 58–9.

[42] ASA, UCH Box, Sister Lucy Mary to Mother Superior, 7 January [1897].

[43] UCHOFF/MIN/6/4, 18 April 1898.

board of the additional nurses, one of the two district nurses, the outdoor uniforms and laundry and the extra servant for the Nurses' Home. It would not pay the £263 12s. 2d. which Sister Cecilia had failed to collect from the paying probationers, nor would they pay for the better-quality food. However, the following year, 1898, after the Sisters had paid the £784 15s 3d., the governors paid for the second district nurse and gave the Sisters £500 for their other expenses.[44]

As well as using the income from the private nurses which the governors thought belonged to them, as the nursing work increased and the governors became less willing to pay for the nurses they already had, Sister Cecilia had added nurses without informing the committee. Mother Superior Mary Augustine sent Sister Cecilia £400 for the Nurses Home, and the governors a cheque for the £784 15s. 3d. they were requesting. She explained that she considered the use of the £500 from the private nursing service for the in-hospital nursing service wrong. Furthermore, she thought Sister Cecilia had been unbusinesslike in several ways: first, in increasing her staff without the hospital's sanction; second, in failing to inform them how much the nursing expenses had increased and how insufficient the hospital payments were, and finally, in remitting some of the paying pupils' fees. However, she wrote:

> The rest of the debt was incurred in the real needs of the hospital nursing staff. And moreover there has been no extravagance in the expenditure but quite the reverse, for it compares favourably with the statistics of other Hospitals.

She recognized that the hospital could not legitimately be expected to pay for what it had not sanctioned, and was therefore sending them the money they demanded.[45]

Although her accounting system was unsophisticated and she was soft-hearted with the paying pupils, Sister Cecilia was not financially incompetent, as has been suggested. Her figures, with some rounding, were the same as those of the hospital governors; she knew precisely what her costs were, what was in accounts receivable and so on. The Sisters covered the hospital's deficit and lent it money, not because they were financially incompetent, but as a part of their charitable work. Like the BNA, however, the All Saints Sisters had reached the limit of their financial ability to maintain adequate nurse staffing and to subsidize hospital operations.

Sister Cecilia may seem a less able person than the immensely competent and self-confident Sister Mary Jones. The sisterhood's deficit weighed so heavily on her that she suffered some kind of nervous breakdown and took protracted sick leave.[46] When she recovered, she asked to be sent to India, but proved too old to start work in such a different climate and soon returned home. She then began

---

[44]    ASA, UCH Box, First and Second Reports of the Special Committee, 22 December 1897 and 28 April 1898; UCH/A1/2/8, 30 March 1898.

[45]    UCHOFF/MIN/6/4, 18 April 1898.

[46]    UCH/A1/2/8, 11 May 1898.

Table 9.1    Cost of nursing per available bed, 1873

| Hospital | Number of available beds | Number of nurses | Number of sisters/ head nurses | Cost of all nursing staff's board and wages (£) | Total cost of nursing & ward cleaning (£) | Proportion of nurses (including Head Nurses) to beds | Total cost of nursing for each available bed |
|---|---|---|---|---|---|---|---|
| St Mary's[a] | 165 | 19 | 7 | 1,520 | 1,520 | 1:6 | £6,15s |
| Charing Cross[a] | 150 | 22 | 5 | 1,014 | 1,014 | 1:5.5 | £6,15s |
| Guy's | 715 | 86 | 20 | 4,934 | 5,220 | 1:6.7 | £7,6s |
| London[b] | 640 | 94 | 16 | 5,418 | 5,992 | 1:5.8 | £9,7s |
| St Bartholomew's[b] | 676 | 81 | 25 | 5,878 | 6,411 | 1:6.37 | £9,9s,8d |
| University College[a] | 150 | 30 | 5 | 1,500[c] | 1,500 | 1:4.28 | £10, |
| St George's | 353 | 54 | 14 | 3,200[d] | 3,650[d] | 1:5.2 | £10,6s |
| St Thomas' | 400 | 75[e] | 13 | 3,960 | 4,500 | No information | £11,5s |
| Middlesex[f] | 320 | 42 | 10 | 3,250 | 3,650 | 1:6.15 | £11,8s |
| King's College | 172 | 42 | 10 | 2000 | 2260 | 1:3.44 | £13,2s,9d |

*Notes*: a. The cost of cleaners (scrubbers/ward women) included in nursing costs.

b. Noted that these costs would shortly increase, at St Bartholomew's due to an increase in wages.

c. Included all female servants in hospital.

d. Included estimates.

e. Included an estimated 30 probationers maintained chiefly at the expense of the Nightingale Fund.

f. Included cost of detached Nurses' Home.

Source: Adapted from 'Nursing Arrangements of the London Hospitals', BMJ, 4 April 1874, p. 461.

what the Sisters called 'the finest part of her life, a life of prayer and quiet service'. The Sisters and nurses who worked under her remembered her as a great lady who ruled everyone, including the Hospital Committee, with a rod of iron. Her nurses especially appreciated the improvements she made in their living quarters, while a later, secular matron thought her letters to the committee demonstrated a very vigorous mind.[47]

In its study of nursing systems in 1874, the *British Medical Journal* did not think that the charge of higher costs for sisterhood nursing was fair. What caused the greater expense was, as the Medical Committee and the Sisters themselves clearly identified, the higher level of medical activity. The *BMJ* concluded: 'The difference in the cost [of nursing] is due solely to the difference in the number of nurses required by the hospital.' This assertion was proved by the fact that the two hospitals with the highest and the lowest costs, King's and Charing Cross, were both nursed by St John's House, as indicated in Table 9.1.

Nevertheless, the *BMJ* pointed out, although the Sisters' *nursing* costs were not high, the *overall* cost for hospitals which they nursed was higher than those operating under the old ward system. It attributed this to the Sisters' higher standards of cleanliness and their insistence on more expensive diets.[48] This was true to a certain extent, but the higher standards of cleanliness and fuller diets were also part of the new medical practice, as was the need for heavier nurse staffing to support the much higher level of medical and surgical activity.

**Religious Issues**

The High Church practices and traditional nuns' habits of the All Saints Sisters, and after 1868, the frequent fallacious identification of St John's House with the High Church, aroused antagonism in the outspoken, violently anti-Catholic members of the English population. There are numerous examples of institutions in London and in the provinces refusing the skilled nursing of the sisterhoods because of these fears of Popery.[49] In the case of Jones's withdrawal from St John's House in 1868, religious issues were paramount.

How little people recognized the 'cost of suffering and anxiety' with which their work was accomplished, Sister Mary Jones exclaimed in 1865. 'I have had many worries, much hard work – constant disappointments – and some sorrows,' she wrote of her work at King's College Hospital[50] – work which the public generally believed could be done by anyone with a kind heart. When Bishop Tait

---

47    ASA, Sister Elspeth Box, 'Notes about Various Sisters,' pp. 39–40, and UCH Box, *The Nurses' League Magazine University College Hospital*, 15/18 (1976): p. 24. We have not been able to locate these letters from Sister Cecilia.

48    *BMJ*, 4 April 1874, pp. 461–2.

49    See, for example, *BMJ,* 11 August, p. 176, and *BMJ*, 8 September 1866, p. 294.

50    BL 47744, fol. 75.

chastised the Sisters for their insistence on their rights to their own religious life, she replied that the Sisters all lamented greatly:

> that the want of any real practical acquaintance with the [nursing] work in which we are engaged, or the difficulties and hindrances under which we have so long patiently striven to carry on that work, has led your Lordship to judge this sisterhood so harshly.

Tait ordered Jones to keep the matter private, so she could not seek advice from friends as to how best to proceed when the Sisters were considering withdrawing from St John's House. He also ordered a secret investigation of the Sisters' High Church practices.[51]

Tait was not atypical in his dealings with St John's House: bishops in general gave the sisterhoods little support. The sisterhoods were new, private enterprises within the Church, and would not be integrated into its polity until the twentieth century. As such, they were not answerable to any ecclesiastical authority; they were independent of the Church hierarchy – an independence which they prized and wished to keep. The bishops' distrust and fear of the sisterhoods, as historian Brian Heeney indicated, stemmed from deeply held views of the place of women in society as well as fears of their High Church leanings. Sisterhoods challenged beliefs about the role of women which men like council member Christopher Wordsworth cherished. He could not conceive of women being placed on an equal footing with men: anything which disturbed woman's complete subordination to man 'weakens her authority, and mars her dignity and beauty'. Historian Susan Mumm described the relationship between bishops and sisterhoods as 'ambivalent, complex and unhappy'. At best, the bishops were cautious and suspicious, and at worst, openly hostile. Most sisterhoods elected their episcopal visitor,[52] but the St John's House constitution made the Bishop of London President of the Council, and that bishop in 1867–68 was openly hostile.

In the case of University College Hospital, the religious issue does not surface in the records after the board's initial hesitation in 1862, perhaps partly because University College was an unsectarian institution and the hospital's board was less concerned with religious issues. When in the 1880s Dissenting groups attacked the All Saints Sisters because they accepted only Anglican probationers, the hospital governors supported the sisterhood. The Dean of the Medical School expressed 'the complete satisfaction of the medical staff with the efficiency of the nursing at the present time'.[53] But more importantly, Mother Harriet Brownlow Byron founded the sisterhood, not a board of Broad Churchmen, and the Sister-in-Charge

[51]  LPA, Tait Papers, vol. 146, fols 3–4, 10–11, and ibid., vol. 145, fols 357–8.

[52]  B. Heeney, *The Women's Movement in the Church of England 1850–1930* (Oxford, 1988), pp. 7–9, 66–7, citation on p. 7; Mumm, *Stolen Daughters, Virgin Mothers*, pp. 137–49.

[53]  UCH/A1/1/3, 8 July 1885.

at University College Hospital reported only to her. In contrast, a group of Broad Churchmen founded St John's House and was the ultimate authority to whom the increasingly High Church Jones reported for the nursing at Charing Cross and King's College Hospitals.

As medieval developments, sisterhoods had an anachronistic aura. Certainly, early historians of nursing thought sisterhoods an outdated form of organization.[54] These medieval connotations may be why historian Sidney Holloway thought the All Saints Sisters were behind the times, reluctant to change their methods and not prepared to accept changes in medical practice. He thought the fact that they did not change their black habits to white until 1898 proved this.[55] His view does not jibe with Sister Agnes Mary's comment that the work had increased enormously in the scientific direction, nor with the fact that in 1897 the Sister Superior was prepared to arrange a washable white dress with short sleeves to replace the Sisters' black woollen habit for all the Sisters.[56] Holloway may have been thinking of modern, sterile operating rooms, but most surgeons only began adopting aseptic techniques in the late 1890s[57] – procedures which created such an increased nursing workload that three new nurses were needed in the operating room. Furthermore, in 1898 the University College Hospital doctors were not overly concerned with the Sisters' black habits. They told the governors that the Sisters only needed to wear white in the operating room and on the obstetrical wards.[58]

## Power Issues

Basic issues of power also came into play in the demise of sisterhood nursing. Many believed the sisterhood's contracts created a separate power base within the hospital, an *imperium in imperio*. The *BMJ* did not consider this a valid complaint. When St John's House and King's College Hospital went to arbitration in 1874, the *BMJ* pointed out that this was the first time such a problem had arisen, although St John's House had been nursing the hospital for 18 years and Charing Cross for six, while the All Saints Sisters had been at University College Hospital for 16 years.[59] Later, however, doctors did come into conflict with the Sisters over their right to appoint nurses and rotate them through the different services. Some doctors complained that as the nurses became more efficient, the sisterhoods withdrew them for their private nursing services (or for their other hospitals) and replaced

---

54    Dock and Stewart, *A Short History of Nursing*, pp. 113–14; Tooley, *The History of Nursing in the British Empire*, p. 89; E.S. Haldane, *The British Nurse in Peace and War* (London, 1923), pp. 99–100.

55    Holloway, 'The All Saints Sisterhood at University College Hospital', p. 153.

56    UCHOFF/MIN/1/4, 17 November 1897.

57    F.F. Cartwright, *The Development of Modern Surgery* (London, 1967), p. 82.

58    UCH/A1/2/8, 22 December 1897, 19 January 1898.

59    *BMJ*, 14 March 1874, pp. 357–8.

them with inexperienced probationers.[60] In 1878, the University College Hospital Medical Committee thought the Sister Superior was changing both Sisters and assistant nurses too often. The doctors wanted the changes negotiated with them beforehand. The new contract in 1878 specified that at least 20 of the 27 nurses whom the sisterhood was to provide must have had more than one year's experience as a hospital nurse.[61] By the mid-1870s, when the Anglican Sisters were losing their monopoly on disciplined and respectable nursing, doctors and hospital boards became less willing to accept the freedom of action and control of their nursing practice which the Sisters had demanded and achieved in the 1850s and 1860s.

In 1874, Sister Superior Caroline Lloyd of St John's House explained the reasons for moving the nurses from ward to ward. She rotated the nurses, and the probationers in particular, from service to service to give them broader clinical experience. At other times, she moved highly competent nurses to wards where she felt a more experienced nurse was needed. Nurses also frequently had to be withdrawn from their wards because of illness or vacation. Some were not strong enough for the men's wards, while others needed a change from one service to another to relieve monotony. Nevertheless, many St John's House nurses had been on the same service or even in the same ward for years. The Sisters and head nurses, as opposed to the ordinary nurses and probationers, were never changed unless one was ill or for some unusual reason.[62]

The right of the sisterhood to appoint the nurses was the point of contention at St John's House in 1874, and again in 1883 when every one of the 35 Sisters resigned and established themselves as a new, independent order, the Nursing Sisters of St John the Divine.[63] The All Saints Sisters did not stand so firmly on their rights, which may be another reason why they lasted longer in the teaching hospital system. Their 1878 contract gave up some of the powers for which St John's House fought so hard. This contract allowed the Sister Superior to select the nurses and female servants, but the managing committee appointed them[64] – an arrangement which had been standard for the matrons in the earlier part of the century and which St John's House refused to accept. But although the All Saints Sisters were generally less assertive than St John's House, they insisted on their right to organize staffing, moving Sisters, nurses and probationers as they saw fit.

On 28 October 1898, on the recommendation of the Medical Committee, the University College Hospital governors passed a resolution that the nursing should be placed under their direct control, not contracted out to an outside authority. The committee acknowledged the heavy debt of gratitude for the many years

---

[60]   Ibid.

[61]   UCH/A1/1/3, 20 March, 1 April, 22 May 1878; UCH/A1/2/4, 4 December 1878.

[62]   LMA/H01/ST/SJ/A39/20, pp. 5–7.

[63]   Moore, *A Zeal for Responsibility*, pp. 101–65; Helmstadter, 'Robert Bentley Todd, St John's House, and the Origins of the Modern Trained Nurse': pp. 315–17.

[64]   UCH/A1/2/4, 18 December 1878.

of devoted service from the Sisters, and said the decision was not due to any shortcomings in their nursing.[65] The hospital's 'Committee and Staff' reinforced this message with a gift of a copy of a painting by Raphael to Sister Celicia, 'In grateful remembrance of their long association with the Sisterhood'.[66] The issue was – as Lord Monkswell, the hospital's treasurer, explained – that the hospital wanted to take the nursing into its own hands as nearly all the London hospitals had already done.[67] Was it a coincidence that this decision was made just when the Sisters realized they could no longer so heavily subsidize the nursing costs at the hospital? While there is no surviving evidence to prove this was the case, it is likely to have been a contributing factor.

The arrangements the hospital governors made for the new secular nursing service in 1899 demonstrate what the hospital considered the real problem in sisterhood nursing. All the nurses whom the Sisters had trained were invited to stay on under the new regime, and both domestic and nursing staffs were to remain at exactly the same number as the Sisters' staff. However, the matron had no power to assign any Sister to any ward without the approval of its medical officers; she could dismiss members of the domestic staff, but could not dismiss nurses – she could only suspend them, while the Hospital Committee reserved the right to dismiss them.[68] In short, while the new matron at University College Hospital was responsible for the nursing care of the patients and the discipline of sisters, nurses and domestic staff – powers which the matrons in the first part of the century did not have – the most significant difference between the All Saints system and the new secular system was that the matron had lost the key power which the old matrons and Sister Mary Jones identified as necessary for efficiency and discipline: the power to appoint and dismiss nurses. It was, in a sense, a return to the ward system.

## Gender Issues

Finally, the Sisters' insistence on running their own nursing service clashed with Victorian beliefs about the proper role of women. Boards of governors were conservative, and not used to working with self-confident, assertive women. Historian Frank Prochaska pointed out that while philanthropy and moral reform were basic parts of woman's mission, the expectation was that these charitable activities would be carried out within the same structure as the family organization, with male boards providing the direction while ladies followed their instructions.[69]

---

[65]   ASA, UCH Box, Lord Monkswell to Sister Superior, 28 October 1898.
[66]   ASA, plaque once attached to the painting.
[67]   UCH/A1/2/8, 5 October, 7 December 1898.
[68]   Ibid.; UCH/A1/2/8, 15 February 1899.
[69]   Prochaska, *Women and Philanthropy*, p. 17.

The exception to this rule was charities which catered only for women or girls.[70] As Shepherd put it in 1856, the sisterhood was an artificial family. In 1857, Anna Jameson, one of the early leaders of the women's movement, stated this implicitly when she wrote that hospitals needed the 'masculine firmness of nerve and strength of understanding' and 'the masculine intellect to rule through power' on the one hand, and on the other, the feminine nature 'to minister through love, soothing and comforting'.[71] Many nineteenth-century women, Prochaska indicated, challenged this approach.[72] None challenged it more directly or effectively than the Anglican Sisters.

But while that challenge resulted in highly efficient nursing services, it also provoked a strong reaction. 'Combining as they did authority and autonomy for women with Anglo-Catholic theology,' Susan Mumm wrote, 'there was something in sisterhoods to offend almost all the taboos of this profoundly paternalistic and fiercely Protestant culture.'[73] When, in 1867, Sister Mary Jones insisted that the Sisters had the right to their own inner life, Bowman, who had supported her so strongly in the struggle with Shepherd, thought her arrogance passed belief.[74] Nursing the ill was a part of woman's sacred mission, but the independence and the professional expertise which the sisterhoods conferred on their members violated the ideal of Victorian womanhood. The Sisters were religious, modest, patient, compassionate, self-sacrificing and attentive to the needs of their nurses, patients and medical staff as the ideal prescribed, but they were not submissive, dependent or naïve. They directed their own nursing services, handled their own finances, expected recognition of their competence and stood up for their rights as an important part of hospital administration.

## Sisterhood Nursing in the Wider Context

While there were frequent, unproven accusations that the Sisters proselytized, in the 1860s other hospitals and the medical press considered their nursing eminently superior. The report of a committee from the Norfolk and Norwich Hospital heavily influenced Charing Cross Hospital's decision to contract with St John's House. In 1866, this committee inspected six London hospitals, the Great Northern (nursed

---

[70]   J. Godden, 'British Models and Colonial Experience: Women's Philanthropy in Late Nineteenth Century Sydney', *Journal of Australian Studies*, 19 (1987): pp. 40–53. An example was the women-controlled Harley Street hospital for women where Florence Nightingale gained further clinical experience, as outlined in Chapter 4.

[71]   A. Jameson, *Sisters of Charity, Catholic and Protestant, and the Communion of Labor* [1857] (Westport, CT, 1976), pp. 173, 177–8.

[72]   Prochaska, *Women and Philanthropy*, p. 17.

[73]   S. Mumm, *All Saints Sisters of the Poor: An Anglican Sisterhood in the 19th Century* (Woodbridge, 2001), p. 1.

[74]   LPA, Tait Papers, vol. 149, fols 243–4.

by deaconesses), King's College, University College, St Bartholomew's, Guy's and St Thomas'. They concluded unanimously that the best nursing was to be found where: firstly, a superior class of persons, preferably unpaid, constantly superintended the wards; secondly, the nurses were properly trained, and thirdly, charwomen did all the menial tasks. University College Hospital, they said, testified to the excellence of the All Saints Sisters' nursing, and the doctors at King's College Hospital considered their nursing the most efficient.[75]

By the 1870s, however, governors at hospitals which the Sisters did not nurse were becoming suspicious of the autonomous Sisters. When the Westminster Hospital reorganized its nursing in 1873, the governors investigated the nursing at 11 different hospitals. They identified the three standard systems: the ward system, the contract system as at the Royal Free and the sisterhoods' three hospitals, and the training institution as implemented at the Liverpool Royal Infirmary. The doctors thought the ward system the least efficient and the most difficult to improve, while the contract system gave far superior results and was 'in many respects highly efficient and satisfactory', but led to conflicts of authority. The Westminster opted for the cheapest system: the training school model.[76]

In 1879, the London Hospital set up a committee to investigate ways of revamping their nursing. Their matron, Miss Swift, was not a nurse, and they were convinced that they needed a trained nurse, more highly qualified technically than the Sisters and able to teach the probationers. They were even more opposed to sisterhood nursing than the men at the Westminster; they did not want a religious Sister nor even someone trained by the Sisters. They would under no circumstances, they said, transfer control of the nursing from the hospital authorities to a lady, no matter how qualified, who was committed to the ideas of the sisterhoods or other associations of that kind. The sisterhoods had shown 'an impatience of control, a determination to share in the government of an institution, and a tendency to interfere with the medical and civil regulations', which only led to chronic discord. 'These are matters of public notoriety,' they declared.[77] The two disputes at King's were both indeed very public, written up in the lay as well as the medical press, but the London Hospital governors misinterpreted the issues. It was the Hospital Committee which was not honouring the contract, rather than the Sisters trying to change hospital rules.

With the one exception of wanting to keep the best nurses on their own wards, doctors in the hospitals where the Sisters nursed had been supportive of the Sisters because of their vast improvements in patient care. Doctors who had not worked with them, however, were wary of the Sisters. Dr Seymour Sharkey, a St Thomas' physician, expressed a standard view in 1880 when he explained

75   *Lancet*, 3 September and 1 October 1864, pp. 272 and 384–5; CCH/MBG, 3 July 1865.
76   LMA/H2/WH/A1/44, 21 January 1873.
77   LH/A9/61, 1 December 1879, January 1880.

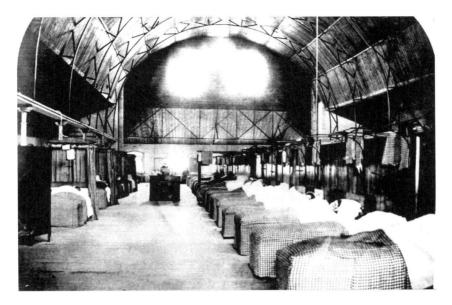

Figure 9.1    Women's Ward at St Thomas' Hospital 1860s. When St. Thomas'
left the old hospital in the Borough in 1862 it moved to smaller
quarters in Surrey Gardens and remained there until the new hospital
in Lambeth was opened in 1871. The building at Surrey Gardens
had originally been designed as a music hall and had only a 200 bed
capacity.

*Source*: By kind permission of the Trustees of the Guy's and St. Thomas' Charity.

that he was very much in favour of the improved nursing which resulted from
more formal training, but he objected strongly to the sisterhood system. He did
not think nursing should be considered a devotional or religious vocation.[78] Yet
it is hard to imagine anyone without a religious commitment who would have
been willing to devote her life to nursing with no pay in the rough, chaotic and
often dangerous hospital world when the Sisters entered it in the 1850s and
1860s. And hospital life was dangerous in two senses: firstly, because of the
undisciplined nature of hospital staffs and patients, and secondly, because of the
contagious morbid emanations from the sick which Victorians believed hospitals
harboured.

Sharkey also disapproved of the Sisters' insistence on directing their own
nursing practice. He argued that it was absurd to say, as the Sisters did, that the
doctor ordered and the nurse executed: 'Is the nurse then to execute in her own
way?', he asked. Nursing was not an independent guild or a separate science, but

---

[78]    S.J. Sharkey, 'Doctors and Nurses', *Nineteenth Century*, 7/40 (1880): pp. 1,091–5.

a very important part of medical treatment, and should be absolutely subordinate to the doctor. In Sharkey's view, the Sisters' insistence on an autonomous nursing service was unworkable. As for the training institution system, he thought it brought little advantage to the parent hospital apart from providing it with a larger stock of nurses to choose from. It perhaps benefited the country more, he admitted, because training schools produced a larger number of nurses, but unless there was a very able lady superintendent, it damaged the hospital, for it necessitated setting aside the ward system. The training institution worked at St Thomas', he said, because the Nightingale Training School had very few probationers, so experienced nurses predominated on the wards, and he declared: 'The basis of the whole organization is the ward system.'[79]

## The Change in the Status of the Teaching Hospitals and their Doctors

When the sisterhoods entered the teaching hospitals in the 1850s and 1860s, the hospitals were public institutions, but as we have shown, they were on the fringes of orderly society. Life within the hospital walls was riotous and disorderly, and staff at all levels moved back and forth freely between hospitals, prisons and reformatories.[80] In 1819, Dr Golding was relieved that St Thomas' was built of red brick with white stone pilasters because that construction differed from most hospitals, which looked like prisons.[81] Because hospitals formed a marginalized area of society, they were more appropriate and less threatening places for ladies to exercise their reforming and ministering mission. Anne Summers pointed out that these institutions were areas where ladies could exercise their motherly moral influence, performing many of the same duties they did in their own homes – duties which were very different from those of the men who ran these institutions,[82] and very different from the work the new nurses would do.

Although the London teaching hospitals were less wealthy by the 1880s, they had dramatically increased in status and were no longer on the periphery of respectable society. While they still catered primarily to the sick poor, they had some middle-class paying patients and had become highly esteemed, known throughout the world as centres of medical research, teaching and prestige. There was also increasing lay respect for the doctors.[83] Furthermore, the sisterhoods had much improved accommodation for their nurses, while St Thomas', the Middlesex, the Westminster, the London and Bart's all had suitable

[79]   Ibid., pp. 1,091–5, 1,103.

[80]   See, for example, UCH/A1/2/1, 29 June 1853; LMA/H01/ST/A106/3k and n.

[81]   Golding, *An Historical Account*, pp. 120–21.

[82]   A. Summers, *Female Lives, Moral States: Women, Religion and Public Life in Britain 1800–1930* (Newbury, Berks., 2000), pp. 13–16.

[83]   LMA/H09/GY/A/225/1, pp. 11–13; Smith, *The People's Health*, pp. 283–4; M.J.D. Roberts, 'The Politics of Professionalization', *Medical History*, 53/1 (2009): pp. 13–14.

Nurses' Homes by 1890. It no longer required the commitment and courage of a religious Sister to take up hospital nursing. As a result, it was easier – at least for the prestigious teaching hospitals – to recruit probationers, and the flood of women into the labour market in the 1880s and 1890s facilitated these hospitals' ability to attract respectable working-class women. It was less easy to attract ladies. Most ladies who took up nursing as a career were downwardly mobile, impecunious women – gentlewomen in the usual terminology of the time – who were looking for a respectable way to support themselves.[84] In order to keep their respectable and – as far as women's work went – well-paying jobs, they were more willing to comply with the more economical but harsher regime which hospital administrators were then setting for nurses.[85] Further, ladies did not have a great deal of choice: respectable alternative occupations did not offer better living and working conditions.[86]

**Conclusion**

In 1874, Sister Caroline Lloyd identified five differences between St John's House nurses and other nurses. St John's House nurses were all Church women and of a respectable character; the Sisters who trained them were thoroughly trained themselves; they were not considered nurses until they had had a year's training; no separate or lower grade of person was used for probationer, assistant or night nurse, and all had a career ladder with promotion based on merit. In a much-quoted statement, she went on to explain:

> every nurse is an object of personal solicitude to the Superior who endeavours to allot to each the work for which she is best fitted .... A St John's House nurse is not regarded by her superiors as a drudge who is to be worked for the convenience of others until she can work no longer and then cast aside as useless, but as a member of a community entitled to sympathy and consideration from those under whom she is placed.[87]

A difference of inestimable significance which Lloyd did not identify but which was to have a profound effect on the future development of nursing was that the religious Sisters themselves worked on the wards, and hence were familiar with

---

[84]   Abel-Smith, *A History of the Nursing Profession*, pp. 29–30; Baly, *Florence Nightingale*, pp. 55–6.
[85]   Helmstadter, 'Building a New Nursing Service', pp. 609, 614, 620–21.
[86]   See, for example, L. Holcombe, *Victorian Ladies at Work* (Hamden, CT, 1973), who gives governesses, shop assistants, teachers, clerks and civil servants as the main occupations open to women. A nurse's salary, with room, board and laundry included, compared relatively well to these livelihoods.
[87]   LMA/H01/ST/SJ/A39/20.

modern nursing practice and able to give the probationers and nurses the benefit of their greater experience as well as moral support. This practice was in marked contrast to the Nightingale system, which, as we will discuss in the next chapter, relied heavily on Home Sisters who were not allowed on the wards. The end of the central system left nursing in the hands of hospital administrators. For these men, good nursing care did not require the same kind of training and respect for the nurses which the religious commitment of the Sisters and the devout evangelicals who ran the British Nursing Association thought basic.

It is not completely unfair to say that hospital boards treated their probationers as drudges to be used or cast aside as useless if they could not keep up to the demanding pace. Historian Sue Hawkins demonstrated that it is a myth that the tremendously high dropout rates in the new training schools were caused by many nurses leaving for that other major career of Victorian women: marriage.[88] Certainly, G.H. Duckworth, who wrote the section on medicine and the law in Charles Booth's multi-volume statistical study of *Life and Labour of the People in London*, was shocked by the toll the training took on the nurses. There was an abundant supply of probationers, he wrote, so hospitals used them for only a few years and then cast them aside and brought in new women. The long hours of work during their training undermined the nurses' health, 'and thus though the hospitals themselves may be well and economically served, the nurses, and ultimately the community as a whole, pay the penalty'. Booth's team, which interviewed many matrons in the late 1880s and early 1890s, wrote that the majority of them reported that no women passed out of 'the hospital mill' unchanged: they were either distinctly better or distinctly worse persons, because the training was a trial as well as instruction.[89] Sister Cecilia thought that nursing took ten years off a woman's life because the work was so hard and the nurses were confined in the hospital, constantly exposed to disease.[90]

Despite their departure from the teaching hospitals, the Sisters left a significant legacy. Under their regime, nurses had gained respectability and could be relied on to give patient care conscientiously. The Sisters' emphasis on training was vindicated: after Wardroper retired from St Thomas' Hospital in 1887 and Mrs Harriet Coster from St George's in 1897, all the matrons in the 12 teaching hospitals were trained nurses. Trained staff were gradually replacing the old untrained sisters and nurses, and although the training varied in quality, the new nurses all had at least the full year's training the Sisters insisted was necessary. Finally, no separate or lower grade of person was used for probationer, nurse or night nurse. Promotion was ostensibly by merit. However, while working-class women certainly became sisters, they had little chance of becoming matron in the teaching hospitals.

---

[88]   Hawkins, *Nursing and Women's Labour*, pp. 148–9.

[89]   C. Booth, *Life and Labour of the People in London*, 2nd Series, 'Industry' (New York, 1970, originally printed 1902–1904), vol. 5, pp. 197–8; ibid., vol. 4, p. 102.

[90]   *PP*, vol. 13 (1890–91), p. 267.

Rather than being anachronisms, it was in large part because they were in advance of their time that the Sisters failed to establish their system as the model for the new nurse. Their recognition of nursing as a specific body of knowledge, their insistence on careful selection of candidates and rigorous training, and their use of merit as the path to promotion were all characteristics of the new professionalism which was developing in the nineteenth century. Even more in advance of their time was their claim to the right of women to hold independent authority and exercise responsibility in the public sphere. This claim lay at the centre of their failure to maintain their position in the teaching hospitals, and once they had left these prestigious institutions, the Sisters were no longer able to influence the development of modern nursing. It would take decades before nurses attempted to reassert their authority within the hospital administrative structure. By then, few remembered that the religious Sisters had previously carved out such a role for hospital nurses.

# Chapter 10

# Conclusion

The title of this book is *Nursing before Nightingale* because perceptions about the origins of modern nursing are so bound up with Florence Nightingale and the nursing school established in her name in 1860 at St Thomas' Hospital. The 'Nightingale nurse', young, trained and dedicated, quickly came to symbolize the modern nurse. However, this outcome was far from a foregone conclusion.

We have demonstrated in this book that there were determined efforts at nursing reform from the early nineteenth century onward. The primary reason for reform was that the new medical therapeutics needed a much more disciplined, conscientious workforce. While the old system threw up occasional outstanding Sisters, hospitals in the early nineteenth century recorded countless complaints about their untrained nursing staff. Our research demonstrates that London Hospital was typical in its 'endless battle keeping their staff in order'.[1] We have also shown the reason for the widespread dissatisfaction. The nursing staff came from a disorderly culture, had no training, worked to largely pre-industrial mores, and, even by the standard of the times, their working hours were long and living conditions poor. Nursing was both exhausting and, as demands on the nurses grew more unrealistic, demoralizing.

Medical practitioners and hospital administrators worked to upgrade the nursing staff so that they could implement the new more successful treatments. Their first solution was the ward system, with a Sister or head nurse in charge of the ward. She received instruction from the doctors and carried out their treatment orders, while the nurses undertook the less skilled menial tasks. The flaw in the system was that it depended on the individual motivation of both the Sisters and the doctors. Some wards were difficult to work and had a high turnover of Sisters, making sustained instruction impossible. Some doctors were dedicated to their hospital practice; others paid cursory attention to their hospital patients, focusing instead on their wealthier, paying patients. It was a 'hit and miss' system; the too many misses continued to jeopardize the advances promised by the new medicine.

Nineteenth-century England was a society where it was taken for granted that Christianity, as exemplified by the state Church, was the foundation of morality. It is not surprising that various efforts to reform nursing sprang from religious roots. The Catholic nursing sisterhoods were widely admired, but could not lead nursing reform in England because of the nineteenth century's virulent anti-Catholicism. The Evangelical Revival produced numerous social reformers, and initially promised the strongest impact on English nursing. The Deaconess Institution at

---

[1]  Heaman, *St Mary's*, p. 25.

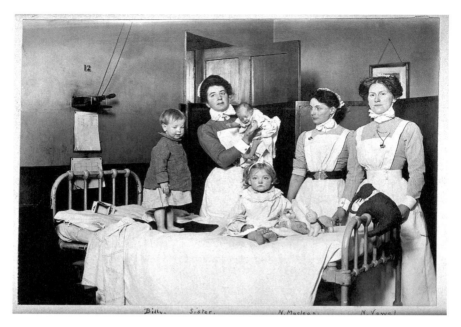

Figure 10.1    The new trained nurses: Sister and nurses at St Bartholomew's
               Hospital, *c*. 1890s. This photograph illustrates well one of the
               favourite themes of the new nursing mystique: the motherly qualities
               of the nurse. The sister holds the baby, while her two assistant
               nurses, indicative of the highly disciplined nature of the new trained
               nurse, stand next to her, ready to receive orders.

*Source*: Wellcome Library, London, by kind permission.

Kaiserswerth in Prussia was one of the first, and most influential, sites of nursing
reform for Protestants. However, its model was not easily adapted to English
conditions. The Quaker prison reformer Elizabeth Fry helped set up the Institution
of Nursing Sisters, but its purpose was to provide domiciliary nurses, and it never
had an agenda to reform hospital nursing. Even Florence Nightingale, when she
attempted to inaugurate a similar system at a hospital in Harley Street in 1853,
failed in her attempt to establish a training school for nurses.

     The breakthrough came from an unlikely source: High Church Anglican
sisterhoods and the Broad Church St John's House. The St John's House
superintendent, Mary Jones, instituted a highly successful nursing system, initially
at King's College Hospital. Like the deaconesses and Catholic Sisters, her nurses
were closely supervised, given clinical and moral training, and exhorted to work
for the love of Christ. It was a highly successful combination, with the hospitals
gaining while the women themselves found a rewarding purpose in life. For

many, it was also an escape from stultifying family life or less congenial work. Yet there was a major flaw: the intense religious conflict of the period and the widespread suspicion among English Protestants that sisterhoods were a cloak for secret Catholic machinations. Jones's move towards High Church practices and her insistence that her Sisters govern their own spiritual life led in 1868 to her withdrawal from St John's House, and also that of the majority of her Sisters. Her successor picked up the pieces, but another dispute with St John's House male governing committee in 1883 led to all 35 Sisters withdrawing and the end of a once highly successful and widely admired nursing sisterhood. By the end of the century, with the withdrawal of the All Saints' Sisters from University College Hospital, there were no longer any nursing Sisters in any of the London teaching hospitals. The evangelical form of the Sisters' central system, the British Nursing Association at the Royal Free Hospital, failed to survive beyond 1884. In this case, inability to raise enough money to subsidize the nursing service was the cause of its disbandment.

The nurses who were engaged by the British government during the Crimean War illustrate the state of nursing in the 1850s. They provide a further indication that it is a myth that Nightingale and her lady nurses revolutionized hospital nursing, and reinforce our argument that clinical skills were central to nursing reform. The secular lady volunteers with no hospital experience were not a success, while the clinically experienced Anglican and Catholic Sisters were invaluable. Some working-class hospital nurses were disasters, while others were excellent, but most had sufficient skills and clinical judgement – including many who had serious personal problems – to ensure they were valued members of the nursing team.

Nightingale's success in the Crimean War paved the way for the Nightingale School of Nursing at St Thomas' Hospital to emerge as the front-runner in nursing reform. It was, in many ways, a most unlikely candidate for such a role. It was run by Sarah Wardroper, who was one of the old-fashioned housekeeper-matrons with no nursing experience. As she grew older, she lost her once outstanding competence and she was too busy to pay much attention to the training the probationers received at the school. Initially, its key medical teacher was Richard Whitfield, who, it increasingly became apparent, had a severe drinking problem. The school came with an elaborate apparatus of teaching and examination of personal and clinical skills, to which, at best, lip service was paid.[2] The intake was small (193 in the first decade) and hand-picked, but still the dropout rate was high: 37.7 per cent during 1860–99.[3] Its nominal head, Florence Nightingale, had little

---

[2]    J. Godden, 'The Power of the Ideal', *International Perspectives in the History of Nursing Conference*, Royal Holloway College, UK, 14–16 September 2010.

[3]    McDonald, *The Nightingale School*, p. 38. Additionally, numerous probationers, such as Lucy Osburn and Maria Machin, were deemed to have completed despite missing months of their year's training.

power to implement her ideals, and refused to visit 'her' school – with one brief exception 22 years after its foundation.

One difference between the sisterhood system and that identified with Nightingale deeply influenced the future development of nursing. The sisterhood system entailed an integration of clinical practice and systematic teaching. The Sisters taught the probationers and worked on the wards where they were exposed to modern practice. In contrast, by 1899 the Nightingale system had not bridged its huge divide between clinical practice and teaching. Realizing that the probationers at St Thomas' were receiving little formal training, in 1872 Nightingale created the position of Home Sister, a nurse who was responsible for the probationers in their off-duty hours, when she gave them some instruction, largely reviewing the doctors' lectures. Practical clinical training was largely left in the hands of the Sisters or head nurses. Many Sisters were not trained in the new system, and few had either the time or the interest to teach.[4] Matron Sarah Wardroper refused to allow the Home Sister on the wards because she thought the Home Sister would undermine the ward discipline.[5] Mary Crossland, who finished training in 1874 and never practised clinically again, became Home Sister in 1875 and remained in the position for 22 years.[6] Miss Crossland 'does not like new ideas', Nightingale wrote in 1896, 'I have never broached to her anything about aseptic or the new ideas about consumption [tuberculosis].'[7] It was the beginning of the system where those who taught nursing were divorced from clinical practice.

There are four main reasons for the unlikely success of the Nightingale School. One was that, however fitfully, the school did value the teaching of clinical skills. Nightingale had learnt this from her time at Kaiserswerth, with Catholic nursing sisterhoods and her close friendship with Mary Jones. The simple fact that nurses needed to be taught clinical skills was accepted: when that was done effectively, nursing practice was transformed.[8]

The second reason for the runaway success of the Nightingale School of Nursing was the phenomenal personal cachet endowed on the school by Florence Nightingale. She was the superstar celebrity of her era, intensely and widely admired for her role nursing during the Crimean War. While she privately despaired of the school, she was so publicly supportive that there was little reason for the public, or nurses, to suspect she was in any way dissatisfied with it. Nightingale captured the public's admiration, and her school and its probationers shared the glory.

---

[4]    See, for example, ibid., pp. 185, 234, 240, 294, 305, 314, 372, 374–5, 453, 458–9, 498; Baly, *Florence Nightingale*, pp. 150–52, 155; Lückes, *Hospital Sisters and their Duties*, p. 15.

[5]    Baly, *Florence Nightingale*, pp. 150–52.

[6]    McDonald, *Florence Nightingale: The Nightingale School*, pp. 894–95.

[7]    BL 47727, fol. 156. Original emphasis.

[8]    J. Godden and C. Helmstadter, 'Woman's Mission and Professional Knowledge', *Social History of Medicine*, 17/2 (2004): p. 169.

The third reason is closely connected to the second: the Nightingale School's adoption of the religious concept of a vocation. Florence Nightingale embodied the self-sacrificing lady so beloved in the Victorian imagination. That successful nursing reform had been dominated by religious sisterhoods helped to transfer the concept of a nursing vocation to a secular context. Along with it came other religious habits: the concept of a probation, the minute examination of character and skills, and the need for an intense community spirit. On a personal level, it was immensely satisfying for many nurses, and provided them with a dedicated purpose in life. The concept of a nursing vocation was seen as the hallmark of the Nightingale School, yet found its most extreme expression outside St Thomas'. Eva Lückes, Matron of the London Hospital from 1880 to 1919, was one of its staunchest proponents. She drove her nurses to service the hospital despite being severely under-staffed and their enduring many of the working conditions of the old untrained nurses, including such practices as 'cox and boxing', with night and day nurses using the same bed.[9] The enthusiasm of the hospitals was understandable: they gained, in one doctor's words, nurses who were 'obedient, efficient and proud of their work'.[10] On the other hand, those nurses who completed their training gained the status of dedicated survivors and were assured that they, in Lückes' words, were not 'ordinary women', but highly special. Perhaps patients gained the most, receiving nursing care which they both admired and trusted.

The fourth reason for the success of the Nightingale School was financial. Like St Thomas' itself, the school had a sound funding basis. It was supported by the Nightingale Fund, put together by donations as a thanksgiving to Florence Nightingale for her work during the Crimean War: its capital amounted to just over £44,000, which, in the early years, ensured a steady income to support the school.[11] It was shrewdly managed by Nightingale's cousin, Henry Bonham-Carter, who was as concerned for the public success of the school as he was to cement his revered cousin's iconic reputation.

What nurses lost most by their identification with the Nightingale School of Nursing, and by the ultimate demise of sisterhood nursing, was an independent base outside their hospital. While Nightingale-style matrons were known as formidable – to the extent that it became a cliché – they had to protect their nurses in an environment where the interests of the hospital, and increasingly the medical staff, predominated. The autonomy of the sisterhoods was tamed. Hospitals harnessed

---

[9]    A.E. Clark-Kennedy, *London Pride: The Story of a Voluntary Hospital* (London, 1979), p. 136.

[10]    Ibid., p. 138.

[11]    Nightingale Fund, *The Nightingale Fund* (London, 1862), p. 3, and *Statements Exhibiting the Voluntary Contributions Received by Miss Nightingale* (London, 1857), HO1/ST/NC/18/02/003, p. 33. Exact conversions to current values are notoriously hazardous, but as a rough guide based on the retail price index, £44,000 was worth approximately £3,000,000 in 2008; <http://www.measuringworth.com/ppoweruk> (accessed 10 July 2011).

for their own purposes their nurses' drive to contribute to social welfare, to lead a purposeful life, and to train in a respectable occupation. St John's House and the efforts of so many throughout the nineteenth century to reform nursing became a footnote, if remembered at all, in history.

The Anglican Sisters' vision of nursing, with its professional autonomy and clinically based education, remains a nursing ideal. The nurses, doctors and hospital administrators who tried to transform an undervalued, disorderly workforce into an effective nursing team were engaged in a prolonged battle lasting most of the nineteenth century. The system we know as Nightingale nursing was the end result, rather than the beginning, of this prolonged and difficult struggle.

# Bibliography

**Manuscript Sources**

All Saints Sisters Archives, Oxford, UK.
Birmingham General Hospital Archives, UK.
Boston University Nursing Archives, USA.
    Nightingale Collection
British Library, London, UK.
    Additional Manuscripts, Nightingale Papers
Charing Cross Hospital Archives, London, UK.
Claydon House Archives, Middle Claydon, Buckinghamshire, UK.
    Nightingale Papers
Columbia University School of Nursing, New York, USA.
    Nightingale Collection
Community of the Sisters of St John the Divine Archives, Birmingham, UK.
Convent of Mercy Archives, Bermondsey, London, UK.
Florence Nightingale Museum, London, UK.
Kaiserswerth Archives, Düsseldorf, Germany
    Nightingale Collection
King's College Archives, London, UK.
    King's College Hospital Records
Lambeth Palace Archives, London, UK.
    Bishop Charles James Blomfield Papers
    Bishop Archibald Campbell Tait Papers
Leeds County Record Office, UK.
    Lady Charlotte Canning Papers
London Hospital Archives, UK.
London Metropolitan Archives, UK.
    Guy's Hospital
    Nightingale Collection
    Nightingale Fund Council Archives
    Nightingale Training School Archives
    St George's Hospital Archives
    St John's House Archives
    St Thomas' Hospital Archives
    Westminster Hospital Archives
Manchester Royal Infirmary Archives, UK.
Pusey House Archives, Oxford, UK.

Nightingale Collection
Royal Free Hospital Archives, London, UK.
Scottish Record Office, Edinburgh, UK.
    Lord Panmure Papers
St Bartholomew's Hospital Archives, London, UK.
St Mary's Hospital Archives, London, UK.
University College London Hospitals NHS Trust Archives, UK.
    Middlesex Hospital Records
    University College Hospital Records
Wellcome Library, London, UK.
    Nightingale Papers
    Queen's Nursing Institute Collection
West Yorkshire Archives, Leeds, UK.
    Leeds General Infirmary Records
Wiltshire County Record Office, Chippenham, UK.
    Pembroke Papers

**Printed Primary Sources**

Atlay, J.B., *Sir Henry Wentworth Acland, Regius Professor of Medicine in the University of Oxford: A Memoir* (London: Smith Elder, 1903).

Beaufort, Emily Anne, Viscountess Strangford, *Hospital Training for Ladies* (London: Harrison, 1874).

Blackwood, Lady Alicia, *A Narrative of Personal Experience and Impressions during a Residence on the Bosphorus during the Crimean War* (London: Hatchard, 1881).

Blizard, William, *Suggestions for the Improvement of Hospitals and Other Charitable Institutions* (London: C. Dilly, Poultry, 1796).

Booth, Charles, *Life and Labour of the People in London*, 2nd Series, 'Industry' [1902–1904] (5 vols, New York: AMS Press, 1970).

Bonham-Carter, Victor (ed.), *Surgeon in the Crimea: The Experiences of George Lawson* (London: Constable, 1968).

Bridgeman, Mother Francis, 'An Account of the Mission of the Sisters of Mercy', in Maria Luddy (ed.), *The Crimean Journals of the Sisters of Mercy 1854–56* (Dublin: Four Courts Press, 2004).

*British Medical Journal* 1854–1900.

Bristowe, J.S., 'How Far Should our Hospitals be Training Schools for Nurses?' (1884) BL/Cup.401.i.7.(8.).

Cheyne, J., 'Medical Report of the Hardwicke Fever Hospital for the Year Ending on the 31st March 1817', *The Dublin Hospital Reports and Communications in Medicine and Surgery*, 1 (1818).

Cooper, Bransby Blake, *The Life of Sir Astley Cooper, bart.* (2 vols, London: J.W. Parker, 1843).

Davis, Elizabeth, *The Autobiography of Elizabeth Davis, a Balaclava Nurse*, ed. Jane Williams (London: Hurst and Blackett, 1857).

Dent, C.T., 'History of Nursing at St. George's Hospital', *St. George's Hospital Gazette*, 2/14 (1894).

Doyle, Sister Mary Aloysius, 'Memories of the Crimea', in Maria Luddy (ed.), *The Crimean Journals of the Sisters of Mercy 1854–56* (Dublin: Four Courts Press, 2004).

Eardley-Wilmot, Frances Augusta, *Memorials of Frederick M. Eardley-Wilmot: Major-General Royal Artillery and Fellow of the Royal Society* (London: William Clowes and Sons, 1879).

E.D. (Emma Durham), *Recollections of a Nurse* (London: Macmillan, 1889).

Ford, John M.T. (ed.), *A Medical Student at St. Thomas' Hospital 1801–1802: The Weekes Family Letters* (London: Wellcome, 1987).

Fry, Katherine and Rachel E. Cresswell (eds), *Memoirs of the Life of Elizabeth Fry* (2 vols, Philadelphia, PA: J.W. Moore, 1848).

Golding, Benjamin, *An Historical Account of the Origin and Progress of St. Thomas's Hospital Southwark* (London: Longman, Hurst, Rees, Orme and Brown, 1819).

Goodman, Margaret, *Experiences of an English Sister of Mercy* (London: Smith Elder, 1862).

Gowing, Timothy, *A Soldier's Experience or A Voice from the Ranks* (Nottingham, privately printed, 1886).

Graves, Robert James, *Clinical Lectures on the Practice of Medicine*, ed. Dr Nelligan [1838] (2 vols, London: New Sydenham Society, 1864).

——, *Clinical Lectures 1834–35 and 1836–37* (London: A. Waldie, 1838).

Mawson, Michael Hargreave (ed.), *Eyewitness in the Crimea: The Crimean War Letters 1854–1856 of Lt. Col. George Frederick Dallas* (London, Stackpole Books, 2001).

Hollingshead, John, *Ragged London in 1861* (London: Smith Elder, 1861).

Jameson, Anna, *Sisters of Charity, Catholic and Protestant, and the Communion of Labor* [1857] (Westport, CT: Hyperion, 1976).

Lucas, R.C., 'In Memorium – Walter Moxon, MD', *Guy's Hospital Reports*, XLIV (1887).

Lückes, Eva C.E., *Hospital Sisters and their Duties* (London: J. and A. Churchill, 1886).

McDonald, Lynn (ed.), *Florence Nightingale on Women, Medicine, Midwifery and Prostitution* (Waterloo, ON: Wilfrid Laurier University Press, 2005).

——, *Florence Nightingale: The Nightingale School* (Waterloo, ON: Wilfrid Laurier University Press, 2009).

*Medical Circular* 1860–61.

*Medical Press and Circular* 1866.

Nightingale, Florence, *Cassandra and Other Selections from Suggestions for Thought*, ed. Mary Poovey [1861] (New York, Pickering and Chatto, 1992).

——, *The Institution of Kaiserswerth on the Rhine* (London: London Ragged Colonial Training School, 1851).

——, 'Introducing Female Nurses into Military Hospitals', in Lucy Ridgely Seymer (ed.), *Selected Writings of Florence Nightingale* (New York: Macmillan, 1954).

——, *Notes on Hospitals* (3rd edn, London: Longman, Green, Longman, Roberts and Green, 1863).

——, *Notes on Nursing: What It Is, and What It Is Not* [1859] (London: Churchill Livingstone, 1980).

Nightingale Fund, *Statements Exhibiting the Voluntary Contributions Received by Miss Nightingale* (London, 1857).

——, *The Nightingale Fund* (London, 1862).

Nicol, Martha, *Ismeer or Smyrna and its British Hospital in 1855* (London: James Madden, 1856).

Overton, John Henry and Elizabeth Wordsworth, *Christopher Wordsworth, Bishop of Lincoln, 1807–85* (London: Rivington, 1888).

Pincoffs, Peter, *Experiences of a Civilian in Eastern Military Hospitals* (London: Williams and Norgate, 1857).

Rappe, Emmy, *'God Bless You My Dear Miss Nightingale': Letters from Emily Carolina Rappe to Florence Nightingale 1867–1870* (Stockholm: Almqvist and Wiksell, 1977).

Rigg, James, *National Education in its Social Conditions and Aspects, and Public Elementary School Education English and Foreign* (London: Strahan, 1873).

Seacole, Mary, *The Wonderful Adventures of Mrs Seacole* (London: James Blackwood, 1857).

Sharkey, Seymour J., 'Doctors and Nurses', *Nineteenth Century*, 7/40 (1880): pp. 1,091–5.

Sister Casualty, 'A Reformation', *St. Bartholomew's League News* (May 1902).

South, John F., *Facts Relating to Hospital Nurses* (London: Richardson Brothers, 1857).

Stanley, Mary, *Hospitals and Sisterhoods* (London: J. Murray, 1854).

Steele, J.C., 'Statistical Account of the Patients Treated in Guy's Hospital', *Guy's Hospital Reports*, 3rd Series, vol. 16 (London, 1871).

Taylor, Fanny, *Eastern Hospitals and English Nurses: The Narrative of Twelve Months Experience in the Hospitals of Koulali and Scutari* (1st edn, 2 vols, London: Hurst and Blackett, 1856, 3rd edn, 1857).

Terrot, S., *Reminiscences of Scutari Hospitals in Winter 1854–55* (Edinburgh: Andrew Stevenson, 1898).

Terton, Alice, *Lights and Shadows in a Hospital* (London: Methuen, 1902).

*The Lancet* 1829–1900.

*The Times* 1848, 1854.

Todd, Robert Bentley, 'Education of Medical Students', *British Magazine*, 11 and 12 (1837).

——, *On the Resources of King's College, London, for Medical Education* (London: J.W. Parker & Son, 1852).

——, *Clinical Lectures on Paralysis, Certain Diseases of the Brain and Other Affections of the Nervous System* (2nd edn, London: Churchill, 1856).

——, *Clinical Lectures on Certain Acute Diseases* (Philadelphia, PA: Churchill, 1860).

*United Kingdom House of Commons Sessional Papers*, 1854–55, 1890–91.

Veitch, Zepherina, *Handbook for Nurses for the Sick* (London: John Churchill & Sons, 1870).

Verney, Sir Harry (ed.), *Florence Nightingale at Harley Street: Her Reports to the Governors of Her Nursing Home 1853–4* (London: J.M. Dent and Sons, 1970).

Warner, Philip (ed.), *The Fields of War: A Young Cavalryman's Crimea Campaign* (London: J. Murray, 1977).

Wilkinson, Joseph G., *Hospital Relief and the Cost of its Administration in the Metropolis* (London: John Elliott, 1868).

Wilks, Samuel, 'In Memorium George Owen Rees, M.D., F.R.S', *Guy's Hospital Reports*, XLVI (1889).


**Secondary Sources**

Abel-Smith, Brian, *A History of the Nursing Profession* (London: Heinemann, 1960).

——, *The Hospitals 1800–1948: A Study in Social Administration in England and Wales* (London: Heinemann, 1964).

Ackroyd, Marcus et al., *Advancing with the Army: Medicine, the Professions and Social Mobility in the British Isles, 1790–1850* (Oxford: Oxford University Press, 2006).

Alexander, Sally, *Women's Work in Nineteenth-century London: A Study of the Years 1820–50* (London: Journeyman, 1983).

Arnstein, Walter L., *Protestant vs. Catholic in Mid-Victorian England: Mr. Newdegate and the Nuns* (Columbia, MO: University of Missouri Press, 1982).

Baly, Monica E., *A History of the Queen's Nursing Institute, 100 Years 1887–1987* (London: Croom Helm, 1987).

——, *Florence Nightingale and the Nursing Legacy* (2nd edn, London: Whurr, 1997).

Bank of England, 'Inflation Calculator', <http://www.bankofengland.co.uk/education/inflation/calculator/flash/index.htm> (accessed 10 July 2011).

Bashford, Alison, *Purity and Pollution: Gender, Embodiment and Victorian Medicine* (New York: St. Martin's Press, 1998).

Baumgart, Winfried, *The Crimean War 1853–1856* (New York: Oxford University Press, 1999).

Best, Geoffrey, *Mid-Victorian Britain 1851–75* (London: Weidenfeld & Nicholson, 1971).

Bolster, Evelyn, *The Sisters of Mercy in the Crimean War* (Cork: Mercier Press, 1964).

Bonham, Valerie, 'Ferard, Elizabeth Catherine (1825–1883)', *Oxford Dictionary of National Biography*, <http://www.oxforddnb.com/view/article/39512> (accessed 10 July 2011).

Bonner, Thomas Neville, *Becoming a Physician: Medical Education in Britain, France, Germany and the United States 1750–1945* (New York: Oxford University Press, 1995).

Bostridge, Mark, *Florence Nightingale: The Making of an Icon* (New York: Farrar, Straus and Giroux, 2008).

Bourne, J.M., *Patronage and Society in Nineteenth-century England* (London: E. Arnold, 1986).

Bryant, Margaret, *The Unexpected Revolution: A Study in the History of the Education of Women and Girls in the Nineteenth Century* (London: University of London Institute of Education, 1979).

Burney, Ian A., 'Medicine in the Age of Reform', in Arthur Burns and Joanna Innes (eds), *Rethinking the Age of Reform: Britain 1780–1850* (Cambridge: Cambridge University Press, 2003).

Buss, W.M. and Vincent Buss, *The Lure of the Stone: The Story of Henrietta Stockdale* (Cape Town: H. Timmins, 1976).

Bynum, W.F., *Science and the Practice of Medicine in the Nineteenth Century* (Cambridge: Cambridge University Press, 1994).

Cameron, H.C., *Mr Guy's Hospital 1726–1948* (London: Longmans, 1954).

Carpenter, Mick, 'Asylum Nursing Before 1914', in Celia Davies (ed.), *Rewriting Nursing History* (Totowa, NJ: Croom Helm, 1980).

Cartwright, Frederick F., 'Nightingales and Eagles', unpublished manuscript.

——, 'The Story of St John's House', *KCH Nurses' League Journal* (1959).

——, *The Development of Modern Surgery* (London: Arthur Barker, 1967).

Chadwick, Owen, *The Victorian Church* (2 vols, 3rd edn, London: A&C Black, 1971).

Clark-Kennedy, A.E., *The London: A Study in the Voluntary Hospital System* (2 vols, London: Pitman Medical, 1963).

——, *London Pride: The Story of a Voluntary Hospital* (London: Hutchinson Benham, 1979).

Collins, Sheila, 'Two Victorian Matrons of the London Hospital', *History of Nursing Society Journal*, 5/2 (1994/95).

Cook, Sir Edward, *The Life of Florence Nightingale* (2 vols, London: Macmillan, 1913).

Craig, Barbara, 'A Guide to Historical Records in London, England and Ontario, Canada c. 1800–c.1950', *Canadian Bulletin of Medical History*, 8 (1991).

Daunton, Claire, *The London Hospital Illustrated: 250 Years* (London: B.T. Batsford, 1990).

Davidoff, Leonore, *The Best Circles: Women and Society in Victorian England* (Totowa, NJ: Rowman and Littlefield, 1973).

Davies, Celia (ed.), *Rewriting Nursing History* (Totowa, NJ: Croom Helm, 1980).

Davison, Graeme, *The Unforgiving Minute: How Australia Learned to Tell Time* (Melbourne: Oxford University Press, 1993).

Dingwall, Robert, Anne Marie Rafferty and Charles Webster, *An Introduction to the Social History of Nursing* (London: Routledge, 1988).

Dock, Lavinia L. and Isabel M. Stewart, *A Short History of Nursing from the Earliest Times to the Present Day* (4th edn, New York: G.P. Putnam's Sons, 1938).

Ehrenreich, Barbara and Deirdre English, *Witches, Midwives, and Nurses* (2nd edn, Old Westbury, NY: Feminist Press, 1973).

Fairman, Julie, *Making Room in the Clinic: Nurse Practitioners and the Evolution of Modern Health Care* (New Brunswick, NJ: Rutgers University Press, 2008).

French, Roger and Andrew Wear (eds), 'Introduction', *British Medicine in an Age of Reform* (London: Routledge, 1991).

Gauldie, Enid, *Cruel Habitations: A History of Working Class Housing 1780–1918* (London: Allen and Unwin, 1974).

Godden, Judith, 'British Models and Colonial Experience: Women's Philanthropy in Late Nineteenth Century Sydney', *Journal of Australian Studies*, 19 (1987).

——, *Lucy Osburn, a Lady Displaced: Florence Nightingale's Envoy to Australia* (Sydney: Sydney University Press, 2006).

——, 'The Power of the Ideal', *International Perspectives in the History of Nursing Conference*, Royal Holloway College, Windsor, UK, 14–16 September 2010.

—— and Carol Helmstadter, 'Woman's Mission and Professional Knowledge', *Social History of Medicine*, 17/2 (2004).

Goldie, Sue (ed.), *Florence Nightingale: Letters from the Crimea 1854–56* (Manchester: Manchester University Press, 1997).

Gregory, Helen, *A Tradition of Care: A History of Nursing at the Royal Brisbane Hospital* (Brisbane: Boolarong Publications, 1988).

Haldane, Elizabeth S., *The British Nurse in Peace and War* (London: John Murray, 1923).

Harrison, Brian, *Drink and the Victorians: The Temperance Question in England 1815–72* (Pittsburgh, PA: University of Pittsburgh Press, 1971).

Hawkins, Sue, *Nursing and Women's Labour in the Nineteenth Century: The Quest for Independence* (New York: Routledge, 2010).

Heaman, E.A., *St Mary's: The History of a London Teaching Hospital* (Montreal: McGill-Queen's University Press, 2003).

Hearnshaw, F.J.C., *Centenary History of King's College London 1828–1928* (London: George C. Harrap, 1929).

Hector, Winifred, *The Work of Mrs. Bedford Fenwick and the Rise of Professional Nursing* (London: Royal College of Nursing, 1973).

——, 'Nursing', in Victor Cornelius Medvei and John L. Thornton (eds), *The Royal Hospital of Saint Bartholomew* (London: St. Bartholomew's Hospital, 1974).

Heeney, Brian, *The Women's Movement in the Church of England 1850–1930* (Oxford: Oxford University Press, 1988).

Helmstadter, Carol, 'Robert Bentley Todd, St. John's House, and the Origins of Modern Nursing', *Bulletin of the History of Medicine*, 67 (1993).

——, 'Doctors and Nurses in the London Teaching Hospitals: Class, Gender, Religion and Professional Expertise 1850–90', *Nursing History Review*, 5 (1997).

——, 'A Real Tone: Professionalizing Nursing in Nineteenth-century London', *Nursing History Review*, 11 (2003).

——, 'Building a New Nursing Service: Respectability and Efficiency in Victorian England', *Albion*, 35/4 (2003).

——, 'Navigating the Straits of the Crimean War', in Sioban Nelson and Anne Marie Rafferty (eds), *Notes on Nightingale* (Ithaca, NY: Cornell University Press, 2010).

Holcombe, Lee, *Victorian Ladies at Work* (Hamden, CT: Archon Books, 1973).

Holloway, S.W.F., 'The All Saints Sisterhood at University College Hospital 1862–99', *Medical History*, 3 (1959).

Hoppen, K. Theodore, *The Mid-Victorian Generation 1846–1886* (Oxford: Oxford University Press, 1998).

Horn, Pamela, *The Rise and Fall of the Victorian Servant* (New York: St. Martin's Press, 1975).

Humble, J.G. and Peter Hansell, *Westminster Hospital 1716–1966* (London: Pitman, 1966).

Huntsman, R.G., Mary Bruin and Deborah Holttum, 'Twixt Candle and Lamp: The Contribution of Elizabeth Fry and the Institution of Nursing Sisters to Nursing Reform', *Medical History*, 46/3 (2002).

Jones, Tod E., *The Broad Church: A Biography of a Movement* (New York: Lexington Books, 2003).

Kinglake, Alexander William, *The Invasion of the Crimea: Its Origin and an Account of its Progress Down to the Death of Lord Raglan* (6 vols, New York: Harper, 1880).

Knight, Alison, 'The Great Nursing Dispute of Guy's Hospital 1879–1880', *International History of Nursing Journal*, 3/1 (1997).

Lawrence, Christopher, 'Democratic, Divine and Heroic: The History and Historiography of Surgery', in Christopher Lawrence (ed.), *Medical Theory, Surgical Practice: Studies in the History of Surgery* (New York: Routledge, 1992).

——, *Medicine in the Making of Modern Britain* (London: Routledge, 1993).

Lawrence, Susan C., *Charitable Knowledge: Pupils and Practitioners in Eighteenth Century London* (Cambridge: Cambridge University Press, 1996).

Libster, Martha M. and Sister Betty Ann McNeil, *Enlightened Charity: The Wholistic Nursing Care, Education and Advices Concerning the Sick of Sister Matilda Coskery 1799–1870* (West Lafayette, IN: Golden Apple, 2009).

Likeman, Janet, *Nursing at University College Hospital, London 1862–1948* (PhD thesis, London: University of London, 2002).

Lloyd, Christopher and Jack S. Coulter (eds), *Medicine and the Navy* (4 vols, Edinburgh: Livingstone, 1963).

London Online, 'Historical Overview of London Population', <http://www.londononline.co.uk/factfile/historical> (accessed 10 July 2011).

Lyle, H. Willoughby, *King's and Some King's Men* (London: Oxford University Press, 1935).

MacDonald, Helen, *Human Remains: Episodes in Human Dissection* (Carlton, Victoria: Melbourne University Press, 2005).

——, 'Procuring Corpses: The English Anatomy Inspectorate 1842–1858', *Medical History*, 53 (2009).

——, *Possessing the Dead* (Carlton, Victoria: Melbourne University Press, 2010).

McBride, Theresa, *The Domestic Revolution: The Modernisation of Household Service in England and France* (London: Holmes Meier, 1976).

McDonald, W.I., 'Jenner, Sir William, first baronet (1815–1898)', *Oxford Dictionary of National Biography*, <http://www.oxforddnb.com/view/article/14754> (accessed 10 July 2011).

Maggs, Christopher, 'Recruitment to Four Provincial Hospitals 1881–1921', in Celia Davies (ed.), *Rewriting Nursing History* (Totowa, NJ: Croom Helm, 1980).

Marcus, Steven, T*he Other Victorians: A Study of Sexuality and Pornography in Mid-nineteenth-century England* (2nd edn, New York: Basic Books, 1985).

Marsh, P.T., *The Victorian Church in Decline: Archbishop Tait and the Church of England 1868–1882* (London: Routledge and Kegan Paul, 1969).

——, 'Tait, Archibald Campbell (1811–82)', *Oxford Dictionary of National Biography*, <http://www.oxforddnb.com/view/article/26917> (accessed 10 July 2011).

Mayhew, Peter, *All Saints: Birth and Growth of a Community* (Oxford: Society of All Saints, 1987).

Merrington, W.R., *University College Hospital and its Medical School: A History* (London: Heinemann, 1976).

Moore, Judith, *A Zeal for Responsibility: The Struggle for Professional Nursing in Victorian England 1868–83* (Athens, GA: University of Georgia Press, 1988).

Moore, Norman, *The History of St. Bartholomew's Hospital* (2 vols, London: C.A. Pearson, 1918).

Mumm, Susan, *Stolen Daughters, Virgin Mothers* (Leicester: University of Leicester Press, 1999).

——, *All Saints Sisters of the Poor: An Anglican Sisterhood in the 19th Century* (Woodbridge: Boydell Press, 2001).

Myers, Pamela, *Building for the Future: A Nursing History 1896 to 1996* (London: St Mary's Convent, 1996).

Nelson, Sioban, *Say Little, Do Much: Nurses, Nuns and Hospitals in the Nineteenth Century* (Philadelphia, PA: University of Pennsylvania Press, 2001).

——, 'The Fork in the Road: Nursing History Versus the History of Nursing?', *Nursing History Review*, 10 (2002).

Newsome, David, *Godliness and Good Learning: Four Studies of a Victorian Ideal* (London: John Murray, 1961).

New York University, <http://medicine.med.nyu.edu/about-us/nyu-hospitals-and-affiliates/bellevue-hospital-center> (accessed 10 July 2011).

Norman, Edward R., *Anti-Catholicism in Victorian England* (New York: Barnes and Noble, 1968).

Nutting, M. Adelaide and Lavinia L. Dock, *A History of Nursing* (4 vols, New York: G.P. Putnam's Sons, 1907–12).

O'Brien, Susan, 'French Nuns in Nineteenth Century England', *Past and Present*, 154 (1997).

O'Donoghue, Jim, Louise Goulding and Grahame Allen, 'Inflation since 1750', *Economic Trends*, 604 (March 2004): pp. 38–46, <http://www.statistics.gov.uk/articles/economic_trends/ET604CPI1750.pdf> (accessed 10 July 2011).

Officer, Lawrence H., 'Purchasing Power of British Pounds from 1264 to Present', *MeasuringWorth* (2009), <http://www.measuringworth.com/ppoweruk> (accessed 10 July 2010).

O'Malley, I.B., *Florence Nightingale 1820–1856: A Study of Her Life Down to the End of the Crimean War* (London: Thornton Butterworth, 1934).

Onions, C.T. (ed.), *Oxford Universal Dictionary* (Oxford: Clarendon Press, 1955).

Paz, D.G., *Anti-Catholicism in Mid-Victorian England* (Palo Alto, CA: Stanford University Press, 1992).

Perkin, Harold, *Origins of Modern English Society* (London: Routledge, 1969).

Peterson, M. Jeanne, *The Medical Profession in Mid-Victorian London* (Berkeley, CA: University of California Press, 1978).

Pfeiffer, Carl J., *The Art and Practice of Western Medicine in the First Half of the Nineteenth Century* (London: McFarland, 1985).

Porter, Roy and Bynum, W.F., 'The Art and Science of Medicine', in W.F. Bynum and Roy Porter (eds), *Companion Encyclopedia of the History of Medicine*, vol. 1 (2 vols, New York: Routledge, 1993).

Prelinger, Catherine M., *Charity, Challenge, and Change: Religious Dimensions of the Mid-nineteenth-century Women's Movement in Germany* (New York: Greenwood Press, 1987).

Price, Richard, *Labour in British Society: An Interpretative History* (London: Croom Helm, 1986).

Prochaska, F.K., *Women and Philanthropy in Nineteenth Century England* (London: Faber, 1988).

Rafferty, Anne Marie, *The Politics of Nursing Knowledge* (London: Routledge, 1996).

Reader, W.J., *Professional Men: The Rise of the Professional Classes in Nineteenth Century England* (London: Weidenfeld and Nicolson, 1966).

Richardson, Ruth, *Death, Dissection and the Destitute* (London: Routledge and Kegan Paul, 1987).

Risse, Guenter B., *Hospital Life in Enlightenment Scotland: Care and Teaching at the Royal Infirmary of Edinburgh* (Cambridge: Cambridge University Press, 1986).

—— and John Harley Warner, 'Reconstructing Clinical Activities: Patient Records in Medical History', *Social History of Medicine*, 5 (1992).

Roberts, M.J.D., *Making English Morals: Voluntary Association and Moral Reform in England, 1787–1886* (Cambridge: Cambridge University Press, 2004).

——, 'The Politics of Professionalization', *Medical History*, 53/1 (2009).

Rosenberg, Charles E., 'Florence Nightingale on Contagion', in Charles E. Rosenberg (ed.), *Healing and History: Essays for George Rosen* (New York: Dawson, 1979), pp. 124–7.

——, 'The Therapeutic Revolution', in Morris J. Vogel and Charles E. Rosenberg, *The Therapeutic Revolution: Essays in the Social History of Medicine* (Philadelphia, PA: University of Pennsylvania, 1979).

Rosner, Lisa, 'The Growth of Medical Education and the Medical Profession', in Irvine Loudon (ed.), *Western Medicine: An Illustrated History* (Oxford: Oxford University Press, 1997).

Ross, J. Cosbie and Ross, John, *A Gifted Touch: A Biography of Agnes Jones* (Worthing, West Sussex: Churchman, 1988).

Roxburgh, Sir Ronald, 'Miss Nightingale and Miss Clough', *Victorian Studies*, 13/1 (1969).

Rule, John, *The Labouring Classes in Early Industrial England, 1750–1850* (London: Longman, 1986).

Schiefen, Richard J., 'Wiseman, Nicholas Patrick Stephen (1802–65)', *Oxford Dictionary of National Biography*, <http://www.oxforddnb.com/index/29/101029791> (accessed 10 July 2011).

Selleck, R.J.W., *James Kay-Shuttleworth: Journey of an Outsider* (Ilford, Essex: Woburn Press, 1994).

Shepherd, John, *The Crimean Doctors: A History of the British Medical Services in the Crimean War* (2 vols, Liverpool: Liverpool University Press, 1991).

Smith, F.B., *The People's Health 1830–1910* (New York: Holmes and Meier, 1979).

——, *Florence Nightingale: Reputation and Power* (Beckenham, Kent: Croom Helm, 1982).

Snow, Stephanie, *Operations without Pain: The Practice and Science of Anesthesia in Victorian Britain* (New York: Palgrave Macmillan, 2006).

Stanley, Peter, *For Fear of Pain: British Surgery 1790–1850* (New York: Rodopi, 2003).

Stanmore, Arthur Hamilton-Gordon, *Sidney Herbert, Lord Herbert of Lea: A Memoir* (2 vols, London: John Murray, 1906).

Stevenson, John, *Popular Disturbances in England 1700–1870* (London: Longman, 1979).

Sticker, D. Anna, *Theodor Fliedner and Nursing* (Düsseldorf: Diakoniewerk Kaiserswerth, 1972).

Sullivan, Mary C. (ed.), *The Friendship of Florence Nightingale and Mary Clare Moore* (Philadelphia, PA: University of Pennsylvania Press, 1999).

Summers, Anne, 'Pride and Prejudice: Ladies and Nurses in the Crimean War', *History Workshop Journal*, 16 (1983).

——, *Angels and Citizens: British Women as Military Nurses 1854–1914* (London: Routledge and Kegan Paul, 1988).

——, 'The Mysterious Demise of Sarah Gamp: The Domiciliary Nurse and her Detractors c. 1830–1860', *Victorian Studies*, 33 (1989).

——, 'The Costs and Benefits of Caring: Nursing Charities c. 1830–c.1860', in Jonathan Barry and Colin Jones (eds), *Medicine and Charity Before the Welfare State* (London: Routledge, 1991).

——, 'Ministering Angels: Victorian Ladies and Nursing Reform', in Gordon Marsden (ed.), *Victorian Values: Personalities and Perspectives in Nineteenth Century Society* (2nd edn, London: Longman, 1998).

——, *Female Lives, Moral States: Women, Religion and Public Life in Britain 1800–1930* (Newbury, Berks.: Threshold Press, 2000).

Sutherland, Gillian, *Elementary Education in the Nineteenth Century* (London: London Historical Association, 1971).

Tennant, Margaret, 'Neill, Elizabeth Grace 1846–1926', *Dictionary of New Zealand Biography*, <http://www.teara.govt.nz/en/biographies/2n5/1> (accessed 10 July 2011).

Thomson, David, *England in the Nineteenth Century: 1815–1914* (London: Penguin, 1950).

Thompson, E.P., 'Time, Work-discipline and Industrial Capitalism', *Past and Present*, 38 (1967).

Thompson, F.M.L., *The Rise of Respectable Society* (London: Fontana, 1988).

Tompson, Richard, *The Charity Commission and the Age of Reform* (Toronto: University of Toronto Press, 1979).

Tooley, Sarah A., *The History of Nursing in the British Empire* (London: H.S. Bousfield, 1906).

Tropp, Asher, *The School Teachers: The Growth of the Teaching Profession in England from 1800 to the Present Day* (Westport, CT: Heinemann, 1977).

Vicinus, Martha, *Independent Women: Work and Community for Single Women 1850–1920* (Chicago, IL: University of Chicago Press, 1985).

Vincent, David, *Literacy and Popular Culture: England 1750–1914* (Cambridge: Cambridge University Press, 1989).

Voth, Joachim, *Time and Work in England 1750–1830* (Oxford: Clarendon Press, 2000).

Waddington, Keir, 'The Nursing Dispute at Guy's Hospital 1879–1880', *Social History of Medicine*, 8 (1995).

Wall, Barbra Mann, *Unlikely Entrepreneurs: Catholic Sisters and the Hospital Marketplace 1865–1925* (Columbus, OH: Ohio State University Press, 2005).

Warner, John Harley, *The Therapeutic Perspective: Medical Practice, Knowledge, and Identity in America 1820–1885* (Cambridge: Cambridge University Press, 1986).

Wear, Andrew, 'The History of Personal Hygiene', in W.F. Bynum and Roy Porter (eds), *Companion Encyclopedia of the History of Medicine*, vol. 2 (2 vols, New York: Routledge, 1993).

Webb, R.K., *Modern England from The Eighteenth Century to the Present* (2nd edn, London: Unwin Hyman, 1980).

White, Eileen, 'The German Hospital – a Unique Story', *History of Nursing Journal*, 3/2 (1990).

Wiener, Martin J., *Reconstructing the Criminal: Culture, Law and Policy in England 1830–1914* (Cambridge: Cambridge University Press, 1990).

Wildman, Stuart, 'Nursing and the Issue of Party in the Church of England: The Case of the Lichfield Diocesan Nursing Association', *Nursing Inquiry*, 16/2 (2009): pp. 94–102.

——, 'Local Nursing Associations in an Age of Nursing Reform: England 1862–1900', *International Perspectives in the History of Nursing Conference*, Royal Holloway College, Windsor, 14–16 September 2010.

Williams, Katherine, 'From Sarah Gamp to Florence Nightingale: A Critical Study of Hospital Nursing Systems from 1840 to 1897', in Celia Davies (ed.), *Rewriting Nursing History* (Totowa, NJ: Croom Helm, 1980).

Williams, Perry, 'Religion, Respectability and the Origins of the Modern Nurse', in Roger French and Andrew Wear (eds), *British Medicine in an Age of Reform* (London: Routledge, 1991).

Williams, Thomas J., *Priscilla Lydia Sellon: The Restorer after Three Centuries of the Religious Life in the English Church* (London: SPCK, 1950).

—— and Allan Walter Campbell, *The Park Village Sisterhood* (London: SPCK, 1965).

Woodham-Smith, Cecil, *Florence Nightingale 1820–1910* (London: Constable, 1950).

Yeo, Geoffrey, *Nursing at Bart's: A History of Nursing Service and Nurse Education at St. Bartholomew's Hospital, London* (London: St Bartholomew and Princess Alexandra and Newham College of Nursing and Midwifery, 1995).

Young, Arlene, 'Entirely a Woman's Question?', *Journal of Victorian Culture*, 13/1 (2008).

# Index